WHAT IS
'Tai Chi'?

of related interest

Alchemy of Pushing Hands
Oleg Tcherne
ISBN 978 1 84819 022 1

Eternal Spring
Taijiquan, Qi Gong, and the Cultivation of
Health, Happiness and Longevity
Michael W. Acton
ISBN 978 1 84819 003 0

Chen
Living Taijiquan in the Classical Style
Master Jan Silberstorff
Translated by Michael Vorwerk
ISBN 978 1 84819 021 4

Tàijíquán
Li Deyin
Foreword by Siu-Fong Evans
ISBN 978 1 84819 004 7

WHAT IS
'Tai Chi'?

Peter A. Gilligan

SINGING DRAGON
LONDON AND PHILADELPHIA

First published in 2010
by Singing Dragon
An imprint of Jessica Kingsley Publishers
116 Pentonville Road
London N1 9JB, UK
and
400 Market Street, Suite 400
Philadelphia, PA 19106, USA

www.singing-dragon.com

Copyright © Peter A. Gilligan 2010

Library of Congress Cataloging in Publication Data
A CIP catalog record for this book is available from the Library of Congress

British Library Cataloguing in Publication Data
A CIP catalogue record for this book is available from the British Library

ISBN 978 1 84819 024 5

Printed and bound in the United States by
Thomson-Shore, 7300 Joy Road, Dexter, MI 48130

Contents

Part I Preliminaries and Preconceptions

The problems of gradings; The problem of cultural
communication; The problem of language; The need for
contextual study; The systems approach; The basic Chinese
world view; Conclusion

Taijiquan as self cultivation; Cultivation; Qi; Yin–Yang; Qi Gong;
Schools of Qi Gong: Internal and external; The use of sensitivity;
The use of intention (will/imagination); The three systems in Qi
Gong; Types of Qi Gong; Jing Gong; Jing-Dong Gong; Dong Gong;
Use of Xin (sensitivity) and Yi (will) in Qi Gong; Summary

Part II Initial Foundation

Part III The Art of Taijiquan

龍騰虎躍
民族精神
徐友題

"It is a delight to all to see the play of tigers and the dragons gamboling in the heavens."

Acknowledgements

Any book is hardly ever the work of a single individual since we are most frequently 'midgets standing on the shoulders of giants'. However, particular individuals deserve mention either as having made contributions without which a particular book would not have been conceived, or whose notable contribution facilitated the book's completion.

Margaret and her colleagues in the original Taijiquan class at DeHavilland College, Welwyn Garden City, deserve special mention. Without Margaret's willingness to ask the questions that no one else would, and her colleagues' willingness and patience to listen to my answers, this book would not even have been conceived.

All my teachers, both Chinese and non-Chinese, most especially the nameless old man in the park in Hong Kong who, despite not sharing a common language, conveyed to me what he called a 'Big Secret' combining Yin–Yang, open and closed, and breathing – an insight that I'm still exploring.

My senior students at the School of Chinese Internal Arts in Belfast, Anne, Colin, Fiona, Harold, Mark and Vivienne, who read and commented on early drafts of the book and have assisted the development of my teaching and the expression of my understanding. All the students I have ever had the privilege of teaching. Without their patience and enthusiasm

I might have succumbed to various suggestions that I 'get a proper job'.

My long-term friends John and Sue Smith who provided invaluable assistance in the polishing of my English text. My illustrators Tony Corey, who created the line diagrams, and Craig Lloyd, the photographer. Andrea Falk of the Wushu Centre, Canada, and TGL Books, for her rigorous and vigorous dissection of the final draft. Tary and Faye Yip of the Deyin Institute of Taijiquan, GB, who encouraged me, as a poor white boy, to persist.

Jessica Kingsley deserves a special mention as my editor. Without her persistence about tweaking and improving the readability of the initial text – the idea for chapter headings is entirely hers – this book would not be nearly as readable as I now hope it is.

Any mistakes are of course entirely my own despite everyone's assistance.

A Note on Romanisation

Pinyin is the system of Romanisation used in this book as this is now the international standard. I make exceptions in certain cases for personal names as these have become familiar in particular forms.

鍛練身心

自強不息

徐友題

"*Ceaseless self-strenthening is required to ensure a healthy mind in a healthy body.*"

What to Expect from this Book

Welcome to my book. Since you have chosen to read a book titled *What is 'Tai Chi'?* I expect that you already have some exposure to the words 'Tai Chi'. Perhaps you have seen a sign advertising a 'Tai Chi' class or you may have started such a class, or have been attending for a while. Alternatively maybe you've read something about 'Tai Chi' where the noted and confirmed health benefits of 'Tai Chi' practice have been mentioned and this has whetted your interest. You might even know a friend, or a member of your family, who does 'Tai Chi'. Maybe your own mum, dad or grandparents do 'Tai Chi' and you think that 'Tai Chi' is something that old people do for their health. 'Tai Chi' seems to be everywhere these days.

So what is this 'Tai Chi'? In that form 'Tai Chi' is something of a Western accident of translation and transmission. We use these words as an abbreviation of a Chinese art called T'ai Chi Ch'uan (Wade-Giles) or Taijiquan (Pinyin). The Wade-Giles form of transliteration is an older form of writing Chinese characters into our contemporary Latin-based script. Pinyin is a more modern system developed and promoted by the government of the People's Republic of China. Pinyin is now becoming the dominant system as it is more likely to be read aloud as something that will sound more or less like the original Chinese. However, when 'Tai Chi' began to attract interest in the West the Wade-Giles system was more common.

Unfortunately Chinese vowels and consonants are moderately unique and any alphabetic transliteration of characters will only be a rough approximation to the actual sounds. In the Wade-Giles system two different Chinese sounds are represented by the letters 'Ch'. One sound was written as a plain Ch while another used Ch', with an apostrophe. The apostrophe is very important in distinguishing between the two sounds. Sadly, to a naive eye their appearance on the page is easily confused and the apostrophe easily gets lost. Pinyin solves this problem by using two different letters from our contemporary alphabet to make the distinction clearer on the page. Instead of Ch and Ch', with the apostrophe, J and Q are used. So Chi becomes Ji and Ch'i becomes Qi. T'ai Chi becomes Taiji in Pinyin and Ch'uan becomes Quan. Hence T'ai Chi Ch'uan is now written Taijiquan.

Pinyin has thrown out the use of the apostrophe altogether because it is confusing and easily lost. This helps eliminate careless Western abbreviated forms such as 'Tai Chi'. A Chinese hearing 'Tai Chi' spoken understands something very different from what the Westerner speaking meant, which does not help mutual understanding at all and has led to more or less amusing misunderstandings. Many Chinese, especially Taijiquan enthusiasts, have now become resigned to this Western mangling of their language. However, the majority of Chinese speakers will not hear what a Westerner means when they say 'Tai Chi'.

With the increasing interest in traditional Chinese medicine (TCM) another Chinese word has also become much more common in the West. That word is Qi, which used to be written as Ch'i with the pesky apostrophe again. The Qi form has even made it into the *Oxford English Dictionary*. When the apostrophe gets lost, as it so often does, Ch'i becomes Chi, which has led many Western 'Tai Chi' players into some confusion. The 'Chi' in 'Tai Chi' is not the same as the Qi in TCM. So what then is the meaning behind the Western accident of 'Tai Chi'?

The Chinese art of Taijiquan is hidden behind the two English words 'Tai Chi'. Taijiquan belongs to a Chinese tradition which started four and a half thousand years ago when the incumbent emperor ordered the people to engage in 'daily dances and exercise to improve the health and strength of the nation'. This long lineage of physical culture makes our Western tradition, which at the most optimistic estimate is little more than three hundred years old, seem quite short and limited by comparison. It is also important to remember the initial and continuing emphasis the Chinese place on 'improving the health and strength of the nation'. The contemporary generic Chinese term for this tradition is Qi Gong, which includes a vast number of different exercises and exercise systems deriving historically from medical, Daoist, Buddhist, Confucian and martial sources. A quote from the second-century Chinese doctor Hua Tuo may serve to encapsulate the vast breadth and depth of Qi Gong. He is reported to have said, 'There is no medicine which may not be replaced by the appropriate exercise. There also is no medicine to substitute for the benefits of regular and healthful exercise.'

What Taijiquan is, in Chinese terms, is one of many ways of self cultivation. It is a particular and unique system of self cultivation developed from the application of Qi Gong to the practice of Wu Shu, usually translated as 'martial art'. So 'Tai Chi' is Qi Gong practised as Wu Shu for the purpose of self cultivation. This would be a short and technically precise answer to your question, 'What is "Tai Chi"?' Unfortunately I doubt that many of my readers will find such an answer either enlightening or informative. It is my self-imposed task to explain that answer, and I hope that after reading this book you will better understand what those words mean.

I shall not be providing a full historical answer to your question. History might inform us about the origin and development of Taijiquan but that does not answer the question about how to do Taijiquan and how to develop your own practice of this endlessly diverse and fascinating Chinese art. However, very, very briefly the history of Taijiquan goes like this. The ultimate origin of Taijiquan is unknown and for those who want to know the exact beginnings of things is likely to remain so. Traditionally Taijiquan is said to have been founded by Zhang Sanfeng, a Chinese culture hero of some note. Facts about him are scarce. The current consensus view is that he was a Daoist priest who lived during the Ming Dynasty, although there are also claims that he lived during the Song or Yuan dynasties some one hundred years earlier. (There is even some suggestion that there were two Daoist priests of historical significance both called Zhang Sanfeng.) Supposedly he was inspired by watching a snake and a crane fighting to create the art of Taijiquan. While this story is of a type common in China, where the origin of something considered important is given a kind of authority by being assigned to the hand of some respected historical figure or another, there is useful information concerning the nature and practice of Taijiquan hidden in this myth. Traditionally Zhang Sanfeng, having invented Taijiquan, passed it to Wang Zong. After him, several generations later, the skill is said to have passed to Wang Zongyue and then to Jiang Fa. Wang Zongyue is the author of the key classical text on Taijiquan, the *Taiji Quan Lun* or *Discussion of Taiji Quan Theory*, which is a defining text for the art.

The next character to emerge historically is Chen Wangting, a ninth-generation family member of Chen village and a retired general. Starting in the 1930s the theory emerged that Chen Wangting personally invented Taijiquan. It was promoted by the communist Chinese government as part of their campaign to empower the Chinese people and remove 'mystical' elements from Chinese history. This theory has become increasingly popular, especially since the 1950s. However, modern research does not support it. Rather the evidence suggests that Jiang Fa taught Chen Wangting while passing through the Chen village. The Chen family art of Taijiquan thus started from this point.

The clear and detailed history of Taijiquan only really can be said to begin with the records and documents of Chen Changxing who was born in 1771 in Chen Jia Go, or Chen village, Henan Province. He taught Taijiquan most of his life and was a tutor in the household of Chen Dehu for many years. Also in Chen Dehu's household was Yang Luchan, who, many years after the death of Changxing, brought Taijiquan to the capital, Beijing, where he gained a great reputation and increased the popularity of Taijiquan considerably. I trace my own teaching back to Yang Luchan who was the great grandfather of Yang Zhenming, also known as Shou-chung, the teacher of Chu King Hung, to whom my own teaching owes the greatest debt. It is the teaching framework of Chu King Hung which forms the core of this book.

Yang Luchan was originally from Yongnian County, Hebei Province, which contains the municipality of Beijing, and to which he returned from the Chen village. Yongnian County is of particular importance in the pre-modern development of Taijiquan, where four famous families lived and shared together their mutual passion for the art of Taijiquan brought from the Chen village by Luchan. These were the Wu (3rd tone), Li, Hao and Yang families, all of whom enthused and practised together, bringing Taijiquan to a further level of development than that of the Chen village. During this phase and in the early days in Beijing the art was unitary;

everyone just practised Taijiquan. It was possible to compare and contrast the particular quirks and emphases of different individuals but at this time they still all practised the art Yang Luchan had brought back with him, which the locals originally called 'Mian Quan', meaning soft fist. It was only after Luchan moved to Beijing that Taiji Quan became the commonly accepted name.

Thus the history of Taijiquan can be divided into several phases: Legendary, Chen village, Yongnian, Beijing and Modern. In the Modern period the art has become subdivided into many styles. In particular the traditional family styles of Chen, Yang, Wu, Hao and Sun plus the officially promoted Chinese government Wu Shu Taijiquan all stand out. This is not to dismiss the existence of several alternative styles, some of which have many practitioners, nor the importance of individuals, followers but not family members, such as Fu Zhongwen and Dong Yingjie.

The shortened version of the Yang form developed by Zheng Manjing (Cheng Man Ch'ing) is very popular, particularly in the USA and Malaysia. The styles developed and promoted by Chen Pan Ling, Liang Tsung Tsai and Kuo Lien Ying are also particularly popular in both the USA and Taiwan. Taijiquan is not the property or the creation of any single individual or family any more than mathematics or music or ball games and sports. Like all these, it is a developed cultural product, created, cherished, refined and expanded by many dedicated, enthusiastic, creative and inspired individuals over many years. Due to the accidents of history and, more recently, deliberate marketing, we may know the names of some of those involved. However, since Taijiquan is both a physical and experiential art that leaves no more permanent trace than do snowflakes melting in the sun and since not all its practitioners will have been literate, we can be sure that the art we have today will also owe a debt to others unknown.

The art of Taijiquan is far from small with many empty hand routines, supplementary trainings and two person practices. It also includes the use of weapons (see Appendix, p.207). What unifies all this diversity is a particular understanding of the principles of body structure and movement and specific methods to cultivate, refine and apply this understanding. In the past Masters and students have recorded their insights and understanding in lists of particular points and poems and songs to inspire and inform both their own practice and that of their students and disciples. In order to truly understand these 'telegrams from history' a deep appreciation of Chinese history and culture is mandatory, since the art of Taijiquan is a particular pinnacle of that rich and diverse culture.

What is 'Tai Chi'?, the title of this book, is the beginning of a journey to further explore the mountain range that is the art of Taijiquan, the great Chinese product that lies hidden behind those two apparently simple words. This book aims to provide the necessary equipment, advice on starting the expeditions and an initial map of the lower hills, to show perhaps a glimpse of the higher peaks in the distance and encourage your own further exploration. The book is divided into three parts: Preliminaries and Preconceptions, Initial Foundation and, finally, The Art of Taijiquan.

Preliminaries and Preconceptions covers a range of potential problems for foreigners approaching the study of a product of a different culture and language. Some of these problems are general ones of interacting with a different language and culture and some are specific to the task in hand in that they may be unique to China. This part also warns of the dangers of preconceptions and introduces some necessary terms. It includes the first three chapters: 1. 'A Punnet of

Problems', 2. 'What's in a Word?' and 3. 'Laying the Martial Ghost'.

Initial Foundation introduces general Qi Gong principles and their application in the art of Taijiquan. It comprises Chapter 4, 'Returning to Nature', Chapter 5, 'Learning How to Learn', and Chapter 6, 'Methods and Techniques'.

The final part, The Art of Taijiquan, discusses in some detail the progression from beginner to intermediate practitioner, pointing out the nested and holistic nature of both the study and practice of this art. It comprises the final two chapters, Chapter 7, 'The Six Secrets', and Chapter 8, 'Practise to Perfection'.

I very much hope you find my little book both informative and enjoyable and I sincerely hope that it will assist you in your understanding and practice of this endlessly fascinating treasure, our gift from the Chinese people.

Preliminaries and Preconceptions

Chapter 1 | A Punnet of Problems

There are many ideas in Taijiquan, and Chinese culture generally, which appear similar to our own but are, in fact, subtly different. To grasp the art of Taijiquan, we also need to understand Chinese medicinal concepts concerning how bodies can be strengthened or weakened. Grasping Chinese medical ideas means coming to grips with Chinese science, which, like all science, cannot be understood without digesting the fundamental concepts of its cultural context, its philosophy, which closes the circle, since Taijiquan both demonstrates and expresses the fundamental Chinese philosophy of Yin and Yang.

Because Taijiquan, in common with many Chinese body arts, is not structured in grades and levels of achievement, it can be difficult to know the order in which things need to be learned, emphasised, taught and practised. There are a number of reasons why the Chinese avoid the ranking and grading system, which originated in Japan, not least because of the historical rivalry between the two nations. In addition, the Chinese are aware of the inevitable flaws in all examination systems (and they should know – they invented examinations as the entry and promotion criteria in the oldest and largest civil service on the planet).

THE PROBLEMS OF GRADINGS

Any examination is a snapshot in time. The most it can reveal is the performance of a candidate at a particular time and in a particular place. The further away that time and place is historically or geographically, the less use is this grading information in the here and now. People change with time and circumstances. One person, having achieved a certain grade, might become complacent and relax, causing a slow decline in performance, down from the examination level. Another might pursue study even more diligently and achieve a current level far beyond that initially recorded.

This is always a problem with examinations. As my grandmother was fond of saying, 'You can't judge a book by its cover', with the examination certificate being a cover for a human being's performance. It is sad, but all too common, that many people, having attained a certain level, then retreat into the fancied safety from personal responsibility that a degree or certificate supposedly affords. Such behaviour can often result in complacency, leading to personal disaster, which can all too easily become more widespread if the practitioner holds a position of social power or responsibility.

In the old days, when physical interpersonal conflict was more common and a knowledge of martial arts was a necessary part of everyday life, complacency about your own or your opponents' level of achievement could very easily lead to the ultimate personal disaster – death. This is a specific martial art problem. Being unduly influenced by an opponent's apparent grade can lead to either over or underestimating their significance. Worse still, focusing on the grade or rank, an abstract characteristic, of your opponent, can blunt your awareness to their actual presence and behaviour in front of you. Survival always depends on accurately assessing the level of threat at the moment of the encounter. Never mind how many belts of whatever colours they have, what are they doing and what does that tell you *now*?

There is a further problem with formal examinations. They tend to be better at assessing theoretical, rather than practical, knowledge. Any test is only ever that – a test. It cannot, by definition, be real. When we used to have engineering apprentice training boards in the UK it was noticed that, as the apprenticeship progressed, performance in regular tests and exams went down while performance on the job went up. As apprentices became better at knowing what to do, they seemed to become worse at expressing this knowledge in a written situation.

There is a difference between 'knowing' and 'understanding' and therein lies a problem. Examinations seem to test 'understanding' but only life tests 'knowing'. 'Knowing' is more than just understanding what to do; it is also being able to do it. It is, if you like, concrete understanding. There is a saying from Taijiquan, 'First in the mind. Then in the body', which encapsulates this fact of life. Understanding seems to be needed first in order for knowledge to be cultivated in action. Later, the knowledge is just there and the person may not be completely aware of what they do. They just do it.

When learning to drive a car, at first we have to concentrate on the pedals and understand what they do. Later we know how to drive, changing gears, braking and accelerating as needed, and all the while carrying on a conversation. Put another way, understanding helps build a bridge between what is currently known and what is to be learnt. Understanding tells us why we do one thing and not another in a particular circumstance. Knowledge just learns this connection, and as long as it works, knowledge is satisfied. Once the link between seeing the circumstance and the best action is strongly established, the theoretical reasons for this link become less important than the fact that it works.

All training systems and schools must be somewhat theoretical, as they are practised alongside, or outside, everyday life. So the use of formal grading systems runs a risk of producing false confidence. In martial arts, this is sloppy thinking that can result in black belts who are bemused that their art was of little or no use to them when they were mugged. In everyday life we have all encountered individuals who rest secure in the knowledge that they have a piece of paper to prove their worth. They can be blissfully, even wilfully, ignorant of the gap between their understanding and their knowledge. Such misplaced confidence can at best be irritating and at worst disastrous.

However, just because we are not convinced of the worth of examination systems does not mean that there is no syllabus. Growth, development and learning are ordered processes that proceed in stages. But here we encounter an initial problem. We are dealing with a cultural product that comes from a different tradition and with a different language to our own. What is 'obvious' to a member of one culture, and easily expressible in their language, may be far from obvious to a member of another culture.

Several attempts have been made to develop classification systems for Taijiquan. A very well-known example is that of Cheng Man Ch'ing, who defined a student's skill in terms of the three powers, Heaven, People and Earth. These come from the Yellow Emperor's classic *Book of Changes*, known as the *I Ching*. He further divided each power into three categories to achieve a total of nine levels. Jou Tsung Hwa uses an adapted form of this system, subdividing each of the three powers into four aspects. These systems are useful to classically educated Chinese, who possess the background to appreciate them. However, for non-Chinese, and indeed non-classically educated Chinese, the style is too poetic, symbolic or allegorical to be very helpful.

THE PROBLEM OF CULTURAL COMMUNICATION

Qi Gong in general and Taijiquan in particular are valued for three main aspects. These are 'ways of self cultivation', 'Shen (spirit) development' and 'work on vitality'. To Westerners these strings of words sound attractive but we really don't know what they mean, since we have no widespread living traditions that are comparable. What is obvious to Chinese is not at all obvious to Westerners. On the other hand, what might be obvious to us might not be so to the Chinese, or might be so obvious as to be insignificant!

The essence of the communication problem lies at the root of classical Chinese thought, in particular in that stream of thought known in the West as Taoism. Westerners have made several mistakes when dealing with different cultures, not least in the arrogant assumption of the inherent superiority of Western thought. This has led to a false division between Confucianism and Taoism being imposed by Western academics. To the Chinese no such essential division exists, and both are considered expressions or applications of the same underlying thought. What we see as Confucian is only the expression of social affairs – Chinese Social Science if you like – whereas what we see as Taoist is the expression of the natural world – Chinese Natural Science.

What is this underlying thought that lies at the base of Chinese philosophical ideas? We could call it Chinese General Systems Theory and not do it any disservice. However, the Chinese would call it Taiji philosophy, Yin–Yang theory or Huang Lao, the Yellow and the Ancient. Its technical terms are Dao, Wuji, Taiji, Yin, Yang, Qi, San Cai (Three Powers), Wu Xing (Five Elements) and specific terms for certain technical areas such as medicine and social relations. At first, these are as obscure to the inexperienced as are the terms of car mechanics to people inexperienced in that particular specialism.

It is by studying concrete examples of a particular discipline that we begin to understand the underlying ideas. In the same way we can learn the meaning of the technical terms of Chinese General Systems Theory. Similarly, a car mechanic learns about the various advantages and disadvantages of different design decisions by working on various types of cars, which furthers his understanding of esoteric ideas such as torque, angular momentum and power to weight ratios. To a trained and experienced engineer, 'torque' is a very useful concept. Personally I have never really been able to get it, which means that mechanics can bamboozle me if they so choose. However, I expect that I could, with sufficient experience, grasp the idea properly.

Similarly, to a classically educated Chinese, the vocabulary of Huang Lao, the Yellow and the Ancient, comes easily and seems to be the most natural and obvious way to talk. This can cause, within Chinese culture, some difficulty in comprehension between the expert and non-expert, on a par with mine when talking to my car mechanic. However, it creates enormous problems when trying to communicate across the cultural divide. The problems are exacerbated when one, or both, sides of the conversation insist on trying to fit these new ideas into their pre-existing cultural and linguistic framework. The folly of this is immense. Something new is something new.

THE PROBLEM OF LANGUAGE

Just to take a little excursion into language, let me tell a Sufi teaching story:

Once there were three men who had only a little money between them. They were all hungry but they could not agree what food to buy. In their hunger and frustration, they came to blows. A passing traveller heard the fighting and offered to settle the dispute by buying something to eat with the money. What's more, the traveller promised that each of the three would be satisfied by the purchase. A little later the traveller returned and the three men fell upon the food with glad cries. 'Angour' shouted one, 'Stafili' another and 'Inab' the third. How could the traveller satisfy all three? What was the food that each called by a different name? The traveller bought a bunch of what we call 'grapes' in English.

In this story, the problem existed because the three men did not consider that it might be possible that they were all talking about the same fruit, simply using different names. Similarly, the three men would have had different words for most everyday things, such being the nature of language.

What happens when the three men come across a new fruit or vegetable that neither they, nor their ancestors, have ever seen before? This actually happened when the so-called New World had the dubious privilege of being 'discovered'. Many new things were brought back to Europe, most bringing their names with them. However, for reasons of national linguistic pride, new words were coined for some of these things. In other cases, these new items kept their names with slight changes in pronunciation and spelling to make them fit into their new language, for example tomato and tobacco are virtually the same in practically all human languages.

From this we can see that, when we meet a stranger with a different language and culture, there are, possibly, two difficulties to overcome. One is that they will use a different sound label to the one we use for a common thing. The second is that they might be talking about something that is so new for us that we have no sound label at all for it. When they are talking about something new to us, there is nothing that we can do except experience that thing directly, and hence learn the new sound's meaning. No amount of language will ever tell you what a tomato is if you have never seen one or eaten one.

THE NEED FOR CONTEXTUAL STUDY

Some things, like names for fruits and vegetables, are easy to move from one cultural context to the next. Give everyone a piece of chocolate and ask them to taste it. 'That' taste, however inexpressible in words, is recognisably different from any other taste so 'That' is now chocolate. The ability to verbalise the experience is not important. Being able to remember and recognise experienced events is what counts; for then a sound label, a word, can be attached to an event.

Part of remembering and recognising has to do with the context of the experienced event, which helps to embed it. Chocolate, as a taste, is contextualised by other tastes and by eating in general. Anyone with experience of small children will know that they go through a stage where everything gets stuck into the mouth, implying a stronger need to taste something rather than know the word for it. But learning a new taste–sound pair is very easy. It was one of the first things any of us ever learned.

Finding words for more abstract experiences than taste can be more difficult. First, we may have to learn how to generate the experience, or have to recognise the several facets within an experience. In Taijiquan there is a technical term, 'Peng'. This is a sound label for a specific form of movement dynamics, which the Chinese would call a particular form type of Qi, or Jing. From a Western perspective, we might call it a particular pattern of accumulating momentum, enchaining the movement of various body parts. Fundamentally, 'Peng' is a type of energy flow in a human body. To assist learning, particularly in the early stages, 'Peng' is attached to a specific posture.

At first, it seems to be the name for the completed posture. In a still photograph, 'Peng', or Ward Off Slantingly Upwards (abbreviated Ward Off), is the completed move. However, Tai Chi is an art and study of energy and movement so the name really describes the move, not its static completion. The still photograph of 'Peng' bears as much relationship to the real 'Peng' as the wavelike ripples on a sandy beach do to the waves of the sea washing in and out.

So, how do we translate 'Peng' in a shorter form than the paragraph above? 'Ward Off' or 'Ward Off Slantingly Upwards' are common translations but these fail to express the idea of 'Peng' as a way of generating energy in movement. The English phrases give some clue to possible applications of 'Peng' in a self-defence context, but only in a very mechanical, not energetic, sense. What is more troublesome is that fixing these phrases as translations of 'Peng' makes further development and understanding more difficult. In the Taijiquan Classics we are told that 'Peng' is the 'father' of all Taijiquan movements and that the whole body has 'Peng'. Substituting 'Ward Off' or 'Ward Off Slantingly Upwards' into these two quotations produces confusion, even gibberish. To make matters even worse, a skilled Taijiquan player is supposed to be able to perform the energy exchanges of 'Peng' and other fundamental movements such as 'Lu', 'Ji' and 'An' without visible movement of the body. If there is not appreciable external movement, we can only be talking about internal energy flows.

Let's take another tack. We can try asking the linguists, who compile dictionaries, what 'Peng' means in Chinese. The short answer is that it does not mean anything in everyday

Chinese. It means 'Peng', what the Taijiquan people do – a technical term. There is an everyday phrase, 'Peng Kai', that describes someone in a crowded place working their way through the press of people. 'Kai' on its own means 'open' as in an action like 'open the door, or window, or box, etc.', but 'Peng' on its own does not exist, except as a technical term in Taijiquan.

So it seems that we cannot translate 'Peng' at all, any more than a Chinese Taijiquan player can to a non-player. 'Peng' is 'Peng' is 'Peng'. It is the technical term for a feature of Taijiquan. It can be very difficult to find adequate words to convey new concepts from a foreign culture. Of course, many people can find such difficulties stimulating and challenging. We are becoming increasingly aware that the Western approach to the world is not entirely satisfactory and there is a search for new and better ways. The existing options need to be refined and/or replaced in the light of new developments and different cultural knowledge.

THE SYSTEMS APPROACH

One of the more recent developments in Western thinking is both the result, and the inspiration, of information technology. This is the product of the confluence of different ideas from mathematics, electronics and cybernetics called General Systems Theory. The applications of General Systems Theory to the natural world alert us to the many problems that technology can create in the environment. The catastrophe of global warming causes more and more people to realise that we are part of the world, whether we like to recognise it or not. Whatever we do has consequences, which can eventually affect us adversely.

Unlike Western thought, classical Chinese thought has always been concerned with systems. In the past we have been inclined to suppose that Chinese ideas were primitive and unsophisticated. This was never true. It is more true to say that our Western ideas have been primitive and unsophisticated in some areas. Unfortunately, the areas in which we were most undeveloped were often those of high development in China. Hence, in trying to simplify these ideas, we mistakenly concluded that the Chinese, not we, were the unsophisticated ones.

We can see how Chinese culture has developed and applied various ideas that we now recognise as similar to new Western ideas. This simultaneously allows us to correct our view of China and to further develop our own realisations. This two-way process of cross-fertilisation will allow a new flowering of ideas, both ancient and modern, Western and Chinese.

THE BASIC CHINESE WORLD VIEW

In the West we see the world as made up of 'things'. Each and every one is alone, unique, different and separated from each other. The universe is a sum of all the things in it. To the Chinese, the only thing in the universe is the universe. All the apparent diversity in the universe is not a collection of separate things but is due to the differentiation or organisation of the universe. A tree or plant can be seen as having different features such as roots, stem, leaves, flowers and seeds. However, a leaf cannot be a separate thing from the plant, nor can the roots be separate from the stem. They can become detached and seem separate, but this is just appearance, not reality. A single leaf detached from its plant is always part of that plant, not a separate thing alone. Taking this just a little further, we realise that a single tree alone still depends on, or is produced by, the earth from which it grows. The soil depends on the planet…and so on and so on until the only single thing is the entire universe. Separate things are a superficial point of view. When everything has a relationship that depends on everything else, then there can only be the one thing – the universe – everything.

Interestingly, this idea of contingency relating everything solves a philosophical problem. Which came first: the chicken or the egg? Well, both are contingent on each other, no chickens, no eggs, and no eggs, no chickens. The boundary of the experienced event is being drawn in an inappropriate place. There is a time sequence that is going: chicken/egg/chicken/egg/chicken/egg/chicken/egg… Chickens and eggs are not separate things. They are two phases of a continuous process, the 'chicken–egg', so the question of which came first is irrelevant. A more reasonable question might be 'Where does the chicken–egg come from?', or 'What is going… chicken/egg/chicken/egg/chicken/egg…?'

The Chinese answer is that the universe is going… chicken/egg/chicken/egg… in much the same way that it is also going …plant/seed/plant/seed, planet/space/planet/space, and people/babies. To simplify and generalise this feature of the cyclical nature of all things, the Chinese used the words Yin and Yang. According to Yin–Yang theory, everything has Yin and Yang, or can be analysed into Yin and Yang. Since Yin and Yang are polar complementary states, or phases of change, there must be a flow from one to another. The Chinese call this flow Qi. So, everything has Qi or, even more fundamentally, everything is Qi. The universe is a Qi web of local Yin–Yang fluctuations. From this perspective, everything can be seen as a wave, which is not a very different view to some emerging in contemporary physics.

This philosophy is so deep rooted and taken for granted in China as being the obvious way things are that it has no special name. Western scholars have tried to label it Taoism, but there is no Chinese philosophy of that name. If pressed, a Chinese might profess allegiance to Huang Lao, the Yellow and the Ancient, after Huang Di and Lao Zi, whose books represent a distilled and clear expression of the 'way things are'. However, the basic ideas of Yin–Yang and Qi are common to all native Chinese thought.

The Chinese view of the world sees it as energy in movement. It is a seething sea of energy, a oneness, indivisible and whole. This energy is the cosmic Qi, the Qi of Universe. Just because it is an indivisible oneness does not mean that it is featureless, undifferentiated or dull. The sea is an appropriate image. It is one, but the waves and currents in it make the surface peak and trough into all sorts of complex patterns. However intricate they become, they are always resolvable into simple patterns of crests and troughs. The complexity of the surface of the sea can be understood and analysed in terms of just two simple features repeating in simple patterns, the crests and troughs of waves of varying frequencies and amplitude.

In the Chinese approach to the world, the universe is energy in complex ebbs, flows and interactions. Objects, people, plants, animals and planets are patterns arising from and embedded in this sea of Qi. The peaks are Yang and the troughs are Yin. Yin and Yang together are sufficient to analyse all this complexity. However complicated the universe is, it can be analysed into a number of simpler Yins and Yangs. This is analogous to the Fourier analysis of complex waveforms into the sum of simple sine waves.

This makes the Chinese approach to understanding 'energetic', as opposed to the 'mechanical' so common in the West. The Western way is to analyse the mechanics and physical dimensions in great detail, while the Chinese look for variation in 'energetic' dimensions. The Chinese would ask about magnitude in terms of intensity, rather than size. We focus on the elements and events in the world; they focus on the relationships.

For a scientific idea to survive we tend to demand that it be useful. In information theory, a bastion of modern science, a rather flip definition of information is that it is any difference that *makes* a difference. Now, in the West, an understanding of the wave nature of everything is becoming more widespread. As the Chinese have been familiar with the concept of the 'waviness' of things and events for much longer than us, we can probably learn a great deal from them.

CONCLUSION

The West has only recently developed theoretical languages to begin to comprehend and translate Chinese scientific ideas. Chinese science is process and function oriented, while Western science has been mostly element and structure oriented. To be able to appreciate Chinese theories more accurately, we had to develop cybernetics, systems theory, information theory, etc. Chinese ideas and concepts have been labelled vague, incoherent and 'superstitious' by us, because our most similar ideas *were* vague, incoherent and 'superstitious'.

The Chinese started with a study of process and function, which led them to develop sciences of complexity, of life and of social science, rather than the physical sciences. Study of the Chinese contributions in these sciences provides two benefits. First, there is intrinsic worth in the Chinese techniques themselves. Finding effective tools and techniques can be much more useful than proving or disproving ideas.

Second, because the 'waviness' of everything is an old idea to the Chinese, we can see in their science how to benefit from applying these ideas more broadly than just in physics and computing.

Only recently has traditional Chinese medicine (TCM) been recognised and explored by the West. The stage has been set for a true interchange between TCM and Western science. Two strands have come together to permit this. First, Chinese prescriptions and treatments definitely work. The Chinese themselves have always been a very practical and empirical people. Their medicine could not have survived as long as it has without actually working. In addition, contemporary experiments have shown that it also can have effects that our medicine cannot achieve.

Therapeutic exercises from TCM, generically called Qi Gong, made a significant contribution to the development of Taijiquan as we know it today. The language of the technical description of TCM is the same language for the technical description of Taijiquan. In Parts II and III of this book, the technical sections, we will develop our understanding of this language. I hope I have established the need for contextual study, so before we move on to technical details the next two chapters of this book will examine Taijiquan in its home context. This concludes Part I: Preliminaries and Preconceptions.

Having examined 'what' Taijiquan is in its home context the three chapters of Part II, Initial Foundation, begin the exploration of 'how' Taijiquan is developed from first principles. Lest we forget, I remind everyone that these are Chinese first principles.

After establishing the foundation of the 'how' of Taijiquan the final two chapters, the third part of this book, represent the technical section, The Art of Taijiquan. In this part the foundation described in the previous chapters is elaborated into the technical details of the performance of the forms and exercises that comprise this art.

The final chapter concludes my sketch of basic and intermediate training and practice of the art of Taijiquan. It also introduces a suggested framework to organise practice and development into a number of overlapping and integrated objectives. Advanced practice, which I will not attempt to elaborate in this book, is shown to be dependent on the necessary accomplishment of establishing a good foundation.

I hope that by the time you reach the end of this book you will have a much clearer idea of the art of Taijiquan: what it is, how it is practised and studied, and why it is that way. If you are a practitioner I hope I may assist you in your practice. Regardless, I hope that this book will serve to explain and clarify the art of Taijiquan.

Chapter 2	# What's in a Word?

TAIJIQUAN AS SELF CULTIVATION

It is difficult sometimes to agree on what Taijiquan is. Is it a martial art? Is it a spiritual discipline? Is it meditation in movement. Is it exercise? Is it therapy? Is it self-defence? Is it preventative medicine? Is it a means to longevity? Some 'Tai Chi' people will say yes to all of these, some to a few, and some to perhaps only one. How can such confusion have developed?

There is a Sufi story about four blind men and an elephant that might be useful here:

> Once there were four blind men who came upon a strange thing. Each of them had touched the strangeness so that he might know what it was. Yet each of them had such different descriptions of what they had touched that they only confused each other when they tried to pool their experience. One said that the thing he had touched was long, thin and whippy with a tuft like a fly whisk or a riding crop. A second agreed that it was long but not thin or whippy at all. Rather, it was quite fat and very mobile like a snake. In fact he had originally thought it was a snake and was unable to understand why the others did not agree with him. The two

others said that it was not long at all. One said it was big and round like a tree or a pillar, while the last thought the other three were all crackers. What he had felt had been big, flat and leathery like an enormous tough fan, although what good such a huge fan could be he had no idea.

The strangeness had a man with it, and he called it an 'elephant'. The blind men were a bit frightened of a man who could associate with such strangeness so they left him and carried on their way, arguing about the strangeness that was 'elephant'.

Of course, to sighted people, what had happened was quite obvious. Each blind man only touched a part of the elephant. One held the trunk, one the tail, one a leg and the last an ear. Perhaps, if they had stayed, the elephant driver might have guided them over his animal, letting them feel how the parts fit together to make the whole animal called 'elephant'.

Taijiquan is a bit like the elephant in the story. The confusion and disagreements result from partial perceptions, cultural misconceptions and historical accidents. What Taijiquan *is* in its own terms of reference is an art of self cultivation. So what is an art of self cultivation?

CULTIVATION

Any farmer knows that a good harvest depends on a number of factors. The quality of the seed is one, but even good seed can be wasted by a poor farmer, while poor seed can be persuaded to a decent yield with good cultivation. Chinese culture is rooted in farming, and some of the earliest traces of the effects of people in China are to be found in water management and agriculture. Most of the land in China is rather poor, and for generations the Chinese farmers have had to work hard to make the most of their resources. The Chinese have learnt that cultivation, making the most of what you've got, is the secret of survival. It is arguable that the Chinese peasant is the best farmer in the world.

With this background, the idea that people are just the passive outcome of the interaction of genetics and environment never really caught on. If the food that you eat is the result of the quality of the seed, the quality of the land and the quality of the effort put into cultivation, then the people that you meet are the result of the quality of their parents, the quality of their food and the quality of the effort put into cultivation.

Cultivation is not something that stops at a certain age. Trees and copses need long-term management, as do irrigation schemes and cities. In the same way, the responsibility for the family farm is passed down from generation to generation, along with the accumulated knowledge of those who have worked the land. With humans, the early cultivation is by the parents. Each person, as they become adult, then inherits responsibility for their own self cultivation.

Some Westerners have difficulty with the idea of self cultivation. They think it sounds anti-social, egotistical and selfish. However, if you want to make your best contribution to other people, how can you do it if you are running on only two or three out of four cylinders? Put another way, how can you expect to do good if you don't feel good?

On top of that, the idea of cultivation doesn't have any fixed end point. If you plant a row of saplings and carefully cultivate them over the years, you will not force each to be the exact copy of the other. Even if you tried, you couldn't. You can only try to ensure that each tree grows up to be the best it can be. Each tree has its unique expression, its individuality, and this is even more so with human beings. Therefore, self cultivation has to be an open-ended activity.

Self cultivation is the art of living – more particularly living *your* own life, not anyone else's.

OK, so Taijiquan is about cultivation, but what do we cultivate and how do we cultivate it? The 'what' is Qi and the 'how', in the case of Taijiquan, is the art of self-defence or Wu Shu. The main aim of self cultivation is to live a calm, unstressed, peaceful and productive life. Since interpersonal conflict is just about the most highly stressed situation most of us can imagine, it provides a good context to study and practise being calm and relaxed. If you can remain calm in the most stressful situations, then you are likely to remain calm most of the time.

We cannot make an exact comparison between Western 'martial art' and the Chinese term Wu Shu. There is a long-standing history of misunderstanding about the study and application of the methods of physical self-defence as practised in China. For a number of reasons the functional application of Taijiquan has been pushed relatively far back in the syllabus. Indeed there are large numbers of 'Tai Chi' practitioners who choose to practise only the famous, slow motion, solo shadow boxing routines. This is perfectly acceptable for individuals, but it contributes to the confusion around the art. It results in players getting stuck in their understanding, development and self cultivation. I shall go into details of the meaning and purpose of Wu Shu later, but for now let us turn to the 'what' of self cultivation and discuss Qi.

QI

Qi is usually translated as 'vital energy' or 'life force'. This is unfortunate and unhelpful since, in European languages and culture, we no longer have any rich and subtle set of concepts

WHAT'S IN A WORD?

to go with the idea of 'life force'. Because to us 'life force' is a vague and romantic notion, we are inclined to believe that Qi is a similarly weak and not very useful idea. This could not be further from the truth. Qi is a fundamental plank of Chinese thought. The role of the Chinese ideas of Yin, Yang and Qi are comparable to that of our ideas of space, time and motion. In fact, space, time and motion would be partial translations of Yin, Yang and Qi. The reason why they are partial is that the Chinese concepts are broader, deeper and more abstractly fundamental than our ideas of space, time and motion. Thus, Qi could be translated as motion but it is a more general term than motion. As the Chinese say, 'Qi is *in* motion, but it is *not* motion.'

YIN–YANG

Imagine the waves on a pool. Peaks are Yang and troughs are Yin. Imagine also that there is a measuring stick somewhere in the pool. As a wave passes it, the stick will measure Yang as the level rises and Yin as it drops. As the level of water on the stick rises and falls, we can see Yang/Yin/Yang/Yin. The Chinese then say that what connects the Yin and the Yang is Qi. It is the 'communication' between the two states. The wave is in movement but the stick does not move.

The 'wave' links the peaks and troughs, so it is the 'communication' between the peaks and troughs, which are Yang and Yin. Qi flows and communicates between Yin and Yang. In modern terms it is both the information and the carrier of the information. A good example of this is modulated radio signals.

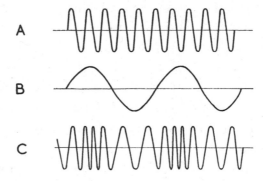

A. Carrier wave, cf. universal Qi; B. Modulating signal, cf. local Qi structure; C. Modulated carrier, cf. specific Qi

QI GONG

Gong means 'hard', 'difficult', or 'work', 'effort'. Therefore, Qi Gong is 'working on the "information and carrier" of everything'. It means to work, study and cultivate Qi. When I asked an old traditional doctor in Beijing about Qi Gong, he twinkled and told me that everything was Qi Gong. He also told me that smiling was a form of Qi Gong, as was acupuncture. He was teasing a little when he said everything was Qi Gong. He knew that my interest was specifically medical and health related, so he answered from the general, not the specific, level, first to tease me and then to test me. Since, from a particular point of view, everything consists only of Qi, the webworks of 'waves' that connect the pattern are the Yin and Yang of phenomena. Thus, all phenomena are the work – Gong – of Qi. Everything is Qi but, since Qi is pattern information producing process and function, it becomes the specific characteristic of living things. Animate matter is distinguished from inanimate matter by its complexity. Living things are highly structured accumulations of elements that differentiate into functions, and have processes that are the patterns of communication between the functions.

From the webwork view, living things are complex knots, concentrations, of Qi. Local Qi structures are like whirlpools and standing waves in the overall flow of a river. Just as the whirlpool has a distinct structure and pattern, despite the continual replacement of its water, so we can talk about the Qi of a particular living thing, despite the seeming transience implied by a 'wavy' reality. The Qi of any living thing is the 'standing wave' or 'whirlpool' that it represents in the ceaselessly 'waving' webwork of Qi that is the universe. This is what the Chinese mean when they talk about specific Qi like 'horse Qi', 'rice Qi', 'human Qi' and so on. In the illustration above 'A' would represent the universal Qi, the background Qi that is the only 'thing' in the universe, 'B' would represent a specific local Qi structure, and 'C' is the resultant of the two combined, the specific Qi, e.g. 'horse Qi', 'rice Qi' and so on.

The Qi analysis can become more refined. Within the 'whirlpool' of Qi, there is an internal structuring or patterning. Whirlpool within whirlpool if you like, so we can talk about heart Qi, lung Qi and so on. But while the Qi structure is the 'cause' or the 'basic reality' of the entity that is alive, the mapping from Qi to anatomy can be difficult. In traditional Chinese medicine (TCM) the 'organs' are functional or process patterning, not simply the anatomical organs of the body's physical structure.

Since Qi analysis is pattern and sub-pattern analysis, a potentially infinite number of 'Qis' are possible, which also makes for a potentially infinite number of Qi Gongs. TCM dictionaries of technical terms list 23 Qis and Qi compounds. As a generic term, 'Qi Gong' refers to a form of therapeutic exercise and an approach to health maintenance and promotion that is unique to China.

What is this exercise system and how does it have its therapeutic effects? We can discover clues in the fact that this method of self cultivation has had different names at different times in history. The current term, Qi Gong, describes the exercise's objective and purpose but tells us little about its practice. The art has had two names in the past, 'Tu Na' and 'Daoyin'. The first means 'inhalation–exhalation', which clearly indicates the importance of breathing in the exercise. However, the second, Daoyin, is the more descriptive and useful.

Dao (Tao) means way, path or guide. Yin is the polar complement of Yang and means to nurture, induce or develop. It is the trough phase before the peaks of expressing, creating or performing, which are Yang. Compound words including Dao, 'ways', are common in China and Chinese areas of influence, so the translation 'way of nurture' is quite common. I prefer 'guiding and inducing' as a more graphic description of the method and purpose.

Thus, Qi Gong is a therapeutic exercise to guide and induce the Qi and it has something to do with breathing. That makes sense since breathing is movement and 'Qi is in movement'. More than simple breathing is implied, since the movements must 'guide and induce' the Qi. The breathing must be exercised.

Since there are potentially infinite Qis, we can also ask which particular Qis are the domain of Qi Gong. Some exercises emphasise and develop 'deep' Qi or 'structural' Qi. This is the aspect of the whirlpool that connects and 'communicates' all the sub-patterns. In Chinese it is 'Zheng Qi', essential Qi. This has two major components. The first is what we might call the Qi 'skeleton' or internal structural pattern. The second is 'integrational' or communicational Qi, that circulates round the body visiting and connecting the 'organs'. In the medical tradition there are also exercises that have been developed, or discovered, that have an impact on specific organs. Usually, the more general Qi cultivation exercises are preferred.

The communication Qi is the Qi of the acupuncturists, the energy that flows in their meridians. It is this component that is of major therapeutic effect. Certain Qi Gong exercises are designed to target specific organs by specifying particular movement patterns. This affects the organ, via the movement's impact on the meridian flow, in the same way that an acupuncturist's needles target organs by affecting meridian flow.

SCHOOLS OF QI GONG: INTERNAL AND EXTERNAL

There are two aspects of Qi Gong that have produced a spectrum of schools and styles. This spectrum is usually described as ranging from external to internal. Very simply put, the difference between them is that the external way is to train movement patterns into the body, while the internal seeks to sense the intrinsic tendencies to move and so evoke movement patterns from the body. The external emphasises structure while the internal *pushes* process. The actual movements may finally become almost indistinguishable, since both develop and express 'Zheng Qi', essential Qi.

It is virtually impossible to separate the two aspects of external and internal in practice, though different schools may emphasise and focus on either one or the other. In order to be successful, one must work on developing posture, or structure (external), and on feeling the moves to guide and develop the Qi (internal). Sometimes students may not notice internal aspects of external schools, or alternatively external aspects of internal schools. Any resulting lack of awareness can degrade practice sufficiently to delay and impair development. In contemporary China the internal–external classification is

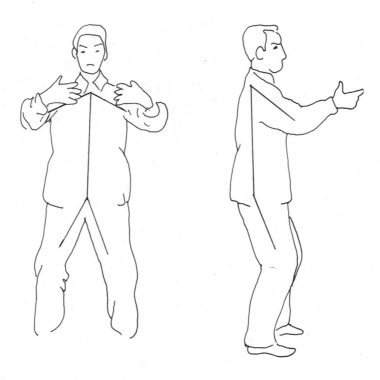

'Bendy Toy' Qi skeleton

beginning to be used less and less. They generally feel that it has outlived its useful life and is now a hindrance rather than a help.

I consider the study of 'skeletal' Qi as a prerequisite to understanding. I think of this as the 'bendy toy' model. When I was young, a new type of toy came onto the market, which consisted of a soft metal wire frame, covered in moulded foam rubber, in the form of a doll. The novelty was that, due to the framework and the pliability of the rubber, the dolls could be moved and posed quite freely. I use this image to encourage people to rectify or correct their posture and structure by focusing on this inner frame. This is working to promote quite specific external effects in terms of spinal alignment, pelvic tilt and limb connection. Although it is expressed in internal imagery, it is an external rebuilding that is desired.

Having achieved this 'bendy toy' external rectification, through mentally guiding the wire frame model from the inside, we move on to Daoyin proper, which is the actual moving. Since Qi is in movement, any movements that are favoured or more likely for a rectified body must be expressions of Qi, in particular the circulating, flowing, communication Qi. Such tendencies to move are the spoor, or tracks, of Qi, the Dao of Daoyin. When we can follow the tendencies and lead them gently into greater and freer expression, we will be nurturing and inducing the Qi in its flowing. Like water flowing over the earth and following irregularities, the way of least resistance, the flow develops and deepens the irregularities to cut streams, rivers and canyons of increasing depth and power.

THE USE OF SENSITIVITY

In order to feel these slight tendencies to move, we must both relax and correct the body so as to reveal them as clearly as possible. To do this, we must use the 'Xin', which can be described as a function, capacity or 'organ'. This is most often translated as 'heart' in the West, since the Qi 'organ' Xin is associated with the anatomical heart. However, since it is a functional organ in the TCM system analysis of a human being, it includes the hardware of the anatomical heart, but is not reduced to merely that thumping muscle.

Xin is 'feeling organ' in the broadest sense. Sensations, perceptions and emotions are all possible because of the Xin. Thus in TCM, many conditions we would call psychological disorders are diagnosed as Xin disorders. These have been

49

poorly translated as 'broken heart' diagnoses and have been used to mock the 'unsophisticated' Chinese. But what these diagnoses signify is the disruption of sensation, perception and emotion with the attendant symptomatic consequences. This parallels a diagnosis of schizophrenia – which incidentally is derived from 'broken head' in Greek.

The Xin in this facet can also be regarded as a mental organ. In certain contexts it is translated as 'mind' instead of 'heart' but this can be confusing since it is not equivalent to what we mean by mind. Xin is 'feeling mind', sensitivity or even sentiment. It is Xin that lets us become aware of the Dao, but we use a different facet for the Yin or nurturing activity.

THE USE OF INTENTION (WILL/ IMAGINATION)

To pursue Daoyin, another part of your mind is needed. The Chinese call this 'Yi' and it is the guiding function. It is intention, imagination, or will. It is the director or goal setter as well as the executor or motive promoter. The Xin finds or detects the tendencies to move. Then the Yi extrapolates them into exercises, which it monitors and directs, subject to the constant feedback provided by the Xin. Hence, there is derived the Chinese proverb that 'the mind (Xin) is the commander of the Qi'.

THE THREE SYSTEMS IN QI GONG

In the practice of Daoyin three systems are interlinked. These are the body, the breathing and the mind, particularly the Xin, sensing, and the Yi, intending, facets.

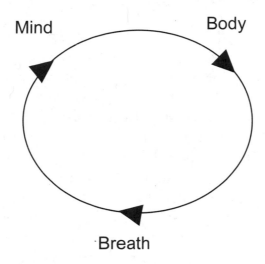

Mind   Body

Breath

The three systems required for Daoyin/Qigong

The mind finds the natural tendencies to move in the body,
its inherent and continual movements. This Dao of movement
is then nurtured and developed. Since the source of these
movements is ultimately the breath, this induces the development of breathing.

When correct, the movements make the body breathe, like
pumping a bellows. The improved breathing relaxes the body
and the mind, improving sensation and thus helping to fine
tune intention. Thus, the mind is nurtured and developed,
strengthening the Xin and the Yi. This affects the body's
moving and, from there, round the body, breath and mind
in a cycle of mutual enhancement. All this movement has an
impact on the Qi since the Qi is in movement. These movements have been called 'dredging the channels' in China, by
analogy with dredging operations to improve irrigation systems. With this dredging and increased capacity, the Qi is
stimulated to develop, hence 'Qi Gong' – work on Qi.

TYPES OF QI GONG

The doctors of TCM identify three main types of Qi Gong. These are Jing Gong, quiescent work, Dong Gong, dynamic work, and Jing-Dong Gong, quiescent/dynamic work.

In the West our emphasis on competitive sport, and the Victorian tradition of 'muscular Christianity', means that we have inherited an approach to physical culture that popularly is seen to reach its peak in the 'no pain, no gain' attitude. This, in Chinese terms, is an extreme form of Dong Gong. For some Westerners that there might be any alternative approach to exercise is almost inconceivable. More sophisticated Western sportspeople are keenly aware that a degree of sensitivity is essential to optimal performance. However, this is not the culturally dominant paradigm.

The Chinese are completely aware of the necessity of a certain degree of unease, or novelty in experience, that is the companion of self cultivation. They speak of 'eating bitter' and the need for some process akin to the 'firing' of wet clay in a kiln to produce a functional pot. But, very characteristically, they point out that pain is nature's way of telling you something is wrong. If your training is truly painful then there is something not right. Change can be disquieting and physical change can be somewhat uncomfortable, or disturbing, if we are not acquainted well with our physical being.

Taijiquan, in its famous, slow motion, 'shadow boxing' routines, is Jing-Dong Gong and this demonstrates the relevance of the classical tag that 'Taijiquan demonstrates stillness in movement'. The complete syllabus of classical Taijiquan includes all three types of Qi Gong. There is Jing Gong: quiescent work, the static posture holding exercises that are 'movement in stillness'. There is Jing-Dong Gong: quiescent/dynamic work, which is the slow forms that are 'stillness in movement'. Then there is Dong Gong: dynamic work, the weapons forms and practices, of which Tai Chi Do or sabre

(Big Knife) is the most dynamic. Depending on the size and weight of the particular 'Big Knife' chosen it can be quite physically demanding.

JING GONG

This is the most important type of Qi Gong for Westerners to understand, particularly if you want to practise Taijiquan or any other 'internal' style. It involves standing, sitting or lying in particular postures. From a Western, dynamic exercise point of view, it can seem that the practitioner is doing nothing, but this is not correct. In Jing Gong practitioners are not doing 'nothing'. They are doing 'not doing'. This may sound as though I am playing word games, but the difference between doing 'nothing' and 'not doing' is vital. If I am doing 'nothing', then I am not working and I am certainly not doing Qi Gong, nor, incidentally, am I meditating, which is also not doing nothing. The Chinese would consider meditation a form of Qi Gong, specifically a type of Jing Gong.

The key word is the word 'Gong', which means 'work', with overtones of hard or difficult. Doing nothing is not 'Gong' or 'work' but rather is daydreaming or falling asleep. In Jing Gong we work to achieve a very particular condition which has two aspects. In the mental aspect we must 'enter quietness' (Ju Ching) while physically we must become 'Song' or 'untied'. This means both a physical and mental release of tension. It is relaxed, but relatively so, not in an absolute sense. It is a physical expression of the idea Taiji, a perfect blend of Yin and Yang.

If you are sunbathing or drowsing in the garden, you will be very Yin, or hyper relaxed. A bodybuilder, posing in a competition, is very Yang, and so tense. In Jing Gong you aim to be equally Yin and Yang – physically Taiji. In this condition the natural movements of living, breathing and heart beating can reverberate through the whole body. Each breath and heart beat works and moves even the tips of the toes and fingers.

There is a sense in which 'you' are not doing anything. When you achieve the correct bodymind condition, the exercise, or work, happens by itself. The 'you' that is not doing anything is your ego or personality. That 'you' is 'Ju Ching', entered into quietness, but your physical 'you', your body, is moving with each breath. The in and out of the breath pumps waves of movement through the body, and so exercises it.

But, and this is an important but, you are not doing 'nothing'. If you believe that the object is to do 'nothing', then you might be too tense and freeze your body so that the movements of breathing do not spread through the body. A fixation on doing 'nothing' can actually prevent you from doing Jing Gong properly. You aim to get out of the way as it were and allow yourself simply to 'be'. By doing 'not doing' with your ego or personality, you release your body to do its natural being. It can then 'work' quietly.

Put another way, in Jing Gong you do not hold a posture rigidly and tensely, which would inhibit or prevent the 'work' of the body developing from its inherent breathing movements. You hold a posture quietly so that it 'works' with each inhale and exhale. This is why it is also called 'movement in stillness'. At first glance, the Jing Gong practitioners are certainly still. They are not moving about actively but, if you observe them, you will see a pulse of movement, a sort of ripple, from the body core to the extremities with each in/out breath cycle. This movement will be very slow when the breathing is slow and so can be difficult to notice. But when correctly done, it is very profound and can result in major effects on the body. So this is Gong or work, but it is quiescent work, Jing Gong.

JING-DONG GONG

This means 'quiescent/dynamic' work and could be regarded as the pinnacle of physical movement. It is most clearly seen in the solo forms of Taijiquan although it is by no means unique or exclusive to this particular art. It is a perfect harmonious blend of quiet and dynamism, whether in the art of Taijiquan or not.

In the solo forms of Taijiquan the player is encouraged to develop 'stillness in movement'. The stillness is for the preservation and development of the Zheng Qi, the essential Qi or Qi structure, the whirlpool or standing wave. The movement is the player's execution of the form with steps, turns, kicks and arm movements. Viewing the universe once again as the flow of a river of Qi, what happens is that a particular whirlpool, with its internal structure of whirlpools, is dancing about in the overall flow of the onrushing stream. Stillness moving.

In order to study this carefully, all schools of Taijiquan have at least one slow motion pattern. This is so the Xin and Yi can operate together to ensure effective Daoyin – guiding and inducing. Slowness alone is not the point. Sensing with the Xin, using that felt image as a director of the intention (Yi) is the essence of Jing-Dong Gong. Moving slowly makes this task much easier, which is why it is commonly found in many Taijiquan schools. However, it is never slow for its own sake. It is only slowness with this purpose and associated internal work that deserves to be called Jing-Dong Gong. In the Tai Chi classics we find the phrase 'slower better', which is often translated as 'the slower, the better' as if slowness was some special accomplishment or virtue in itself. I would suggest a slightly different slant along the lines of 'the better one is, the slower may you go'.

The whirlpool can drift gently through a number of different locations while retaining its internal structure and consistency, its stillness, or it can move rapidly from place to place. Moving rapidly may make retaining internal structure more difficult, and so the 'stillness' in movement can be lost, but this does not mean that the 'dynamic' part of Jing-Dong Gong has any absolute ceiling on it. Even in very limited circumstances, if you retain your stillness, you have much greater opportunities for development. Also you learn to cultivate your capacity to retain your stillness in a greater diversity of conditions.

In Taijiquan, Chen style is noted for its forms containing fast movements. This has led to confusion among some Taijiquan players and observers, who mistakenly believe that all Taijiquan is performed slowly. Indeed, it is wrongly thought that Chen style is the only style with such fast movements. These fast moves aim to demonstrate and express what is technically called 'Fa Jin' or sometimes 'Fa Qi', which is a legitimate facet of Jing-Dong Gong.

DONG GONG

This is the physical education/competitive sport style of exercise which is almost exclusive in Western culture. It is characterised by goal setting and achievement: Win the game. Run faster – cut your times down. Get stronger – lift progressively heavier and heavier weights and so forth. To borrow the title of the film of the 1936 Munich Olympics it is 'The Triumph of the Will'. In Chinese terms it is almost exclusively under the domain of the Yi. The contribution of the Xin is virtually non-existent. Unsurprisingly this disengagement of the Xin contributes to many accidents during training which may compromise life and work outside the training domain.

More sophisticated Western athletes do appreciate the importance of sensitivity in producing excellence. Unfortunately popular physical culture is not yet as sophisticated as these elite athletes. In terms of physical culture the Western tradition is relatively young. Only in the late eighteenth and then the nineteenth century has there been much of a Western tradition of organised physical education. Conversely, in China nearly 4,000 years ago the reigning emperor, concerned at the physical condition of his subjects, issued a decree mandating daily engagement by the populace in 'dancing and exercise to build up the health of the nation'. As a result the broad mass of the Chinese populace now has an extensive historical experience of exercise as a means to maintaining their health and fitness life long.

USE OF XIN (SENSITIVITY) AND YI (WILL) IN QI GONG

One way of looking at these three types of Qi Gong is by comparing the relative contributions of Xin (feeling or sensitivity) and Yi (intention or will).

Jing Gong is mostly Xin. The Yi should be primarily concerned with not interfering with the natural movements or work of the quiet body. The Yi schools itself not to try too hard, neither freezing the body into rigidity nor trying to rush the development of the natural movements that spread from the core breathing movements. The Yi enters 'Ju Ching': 'soft essence' or quietude.

Dong Gong is mostly Yi, as it is the practitioner's will that is primary. The Xin or sensitivity can, in extreme cases, be completely ignored, as when a runner 'goes through the wall'. Personally, I regard such self abuse as only acceptable in conditions of extreme urgency, not as a normal or usual part of exercise. By all means run the risk of permanent damage 'going through the wall' if you are a runner carrying urgently needed and essential medical supplies. But it is foolish on a regular training basis.

Jing-Dong Gong is a blend or balance of both Xin and Yi. Feeling (Xin) is primary as it supplies the information to the will (Yi), which then guides movement according to the principle of Daoyin (guiding and inducing). Traditional Chinese medicine makes much of 'mother–child' relationships. Yi is considered to be the 'child' of Xin.

SUMMARY

Taijiquan can be considered an art of self cultivation. From this it follows that self cultivation, via Qi cultivation, is a form of Qi Gong. We have discussed the concept of Qi as the most fundamental aspect of the universe, the communication between the two states of Yin and Yang. Qi Gong, working on Qi, refers to a form of therapeutic exercise, and is also referred to as a means of self cultivation. It can be followed for more instrumental reasons than the open-ended abstraction of self cultivation, i.e. for health problems, relaxation, exercise, pleasure and so on. In order to allow the natural tendencies to movement within the body, it is necessary to work on developing both the external structure and also the use of sensitivity, Xin, and intention, Yi. The three types of Qi Gong have been explored, with an explanation of their different emphases.

Chapter 3	# Laying the Martial Ghost

There is one topic within the Taijiquan community, particularly in the West, that produces such a degree of debate, acrimony, vilification and confusion that I am going to devote a whole chapter to elaborating my understanding. This is the question of Taijiquan as a martial art and/or a system of physical self-defence. For me, it is unquestionable that it is a system of self-defence. I am also more than happy to call it Wu Shu and/or Gong Fu in Chinese. However, neither of these terms can be translated as the English words 'martial art'.

TAIJIQUAN AS SELF-DEFENCE

Life is dangerous. Life can frequently be nasty, brutish and short. Any individual organism must be continuously engaged in dealing with these consequences of being alive. To that extent, being alive is evidence of the continual success of self-defence. Every breath you take is an act of self-defence. If you don't believe me, stop breathing and see what happens. To be alive at all is to continuously defend yourself, to defend and maintain your particular and unique knot of Qi in all the ebbs and flows of the Qi of the universe.

Self cultivation works to maintain, preserve and develop personal Qi. With abundant Qi, radiant health is possible. To be healthy does not mean simply the absence of any current dis-ease. It means functioning at your best at all levels, from the molecular upwards. It means being actively resistant to damage from external influences.

On his deathbed Louis Pasteur, one of the founders of modern medicine, said about external influences, germs, 'Le germe n'est rien, c'est le terrain qui est tout' ('The germ is nothing, the soil is everything'). Your personal Qi, the structured whirlpool of Qi within the Qi of universe, is the 'soil' that Pasteur was talking about. Its quality is what determines if germs get a foothold. Its quality also determines what, if any, other ill effects are experienced. By self cultivation, it is defended by ensuring that nothing that is not harmonious, or relevant, can affect its organisation. So, from there it follows that self cultivation, in the sense of Qi cultivation, is also self-defence, in the sense of staying alive. In modern terms we might speak of signal-to-noise ratios. Self cultivation works by striving to maintain a good clear signal. Its practice actively reinforces the signal and reduces noise to a minimum.

Of course some people will say that I am just playing word games again. I don't think I am. How many self-defence, or martial art, systems neglect to emphasise the importance of being healthy? How many of them claim that they will also improve your health? It is very difficult to fight off multiple attackers with a bad back, a touch of sciatica or double pneumonia. Long before we need to consider the attacks of deranged human beings, these other dangers have to be dealt with. In thinking strategically we must never take anything for granted, nor must we neglect to consider our lines of support.

Taijiquan, in common with much Chinese thought, uses the idea of San Cai (three powers) to organise and memorise its teachings. Many teaching tags have three elements.

What is the purpose of Taijiquan?

- the prolongation/husbandry/cultivation of life
- the rejuvenation of mind and body
- the prevention of senility.

What is the outcome of Taijiquan practice?

- the flexibility of a child
- the constitution of a lumberjack
- the tranquillity of a sage.

What are the levels of self-defence in Taijiquan?

- the defence against dis-ease
- the defence against ill people
- the defence against the sick state.

The last one is easier in Chinese where the three disturbances come across as the same thing, but at the personal, interpersonal and the social levels. The idea of the defence against 'bad' or 'sick' political organisations is the most important for an understanding of Wu Shu, frequently translated as martial art.

SELF-DEFENCE AND MARTIAL ART

I know of one teacher who claims that Taijiquan has 'grown out of' martial art. The suggestion seems to be that Taijiquan is now beyond 'that sort of thing'. Looking at some of the more ethereal schools of Tai Chi, we might be tempted to ask quite what it is they are supposed to have grown into.

There are schools where fighting is very important and their practice is assertively martial. Sadly, in these fighting schools there is often a sense of something missing. Their art does not seem particularly internal, or as mysterious as their reputation might lead us to expect. They may be good fighters, but reading the classics and stories of past Masters makes us wonder if this can really be the 'supreme ultimate boxing' of the past.

This confusion is the product of arrogance on both sides. Both these schools share the single-minded arrogance of the Western point of view. They are emphasising one element at the expense of the other and thereby missing the essence of Taiji, which comprises both. It stems from our Western assurance that our mental frameworks are the ultimate in sophistication and so we tend to approach everything from a position of smug self-confidence. The bankruptcy of our ideas and ways of dealing with the world are becoming increasingly clear, both personally and globally, hence the interest in other approaches like Taijiquan. However, this complacency often blinkers us too much to allow an open mind to the teachings of another culture and world view. We know that we need something to either shore up or replace our current understanding and way of living. Unfortunately, we too often try to fit the new ideas into the boundaries of our existing framework. This usually results in a faulty transmission of the original idea. It can become a crude and simplified parody.

The polarity between combative and non-combative Taijiquan players is just such a parody. It shatters the art of Taijiquan into its two components, Yin and Yang, demonstrating a complete failure to understand Taiji itself, which is both Yin and Yang. As I have said before, this is due to a misunderstanding of what the original Masters meant by particular words, in this case 'Wu Shu' translated as 'martial art'.

In order to be able to really appreciate what the old Masters meant, we must do more than just copy movements and read translations of classical texts. As it says in the Taijiquan classics, 'To learn something good you have to use your mind a little.' We must understand the art in its own terms and context, not ours. As outsiders we must also study the background. Because of the differences between Chinese and Western cultures, we need to study the derivations and background of both languages in order to understand where these misconceptions arise.

WU AND MARTIAL ARE NOT THE SAME

Take the word 'martial'. It is a derivative of Roman 'Mars', the god of war. To us it means 'war related' in a Roman sense with all that implies: hierarchically organised, authoritarian, with soldiers obeying orders and human beings reduced to elements, considered as merely battle fodder, individually insignificant and needing to bolster their esteem through posturing, posing and displays of machismo.

With all those undesirable facets, it is understandable that some people would prefer to reject the 'martial art' aspect of Taijiquan. The trouble is that the Chinese character 'Wu', which is usually translated as 'martial', does not mean any of that. Therefore, the etherealists are simply rejecting their own projections and fears. On the other hand, those Taijiquan players who are busy being 'martial' in the Roman sense of armies and soldiers are not learning anything either. They are just acting out our Western mythologies.

So what does 'Wu' mean? What do the Masters mean when they call Taijiquan 'Wu Shu'? Like many Chinese characters

'Wu' is an ideograph, or idea picture, composed of two simpler pictures. 'Wu' is a compound of the pictures for 'stop' and 'spear'. So, 'Wu' does not mean anything like 'martial' in the Roman sense and indeed, if anything, it means virtually the opposite. 'Wu Shu' is the 'art of stopping the spear'. If we take the 'spear' to represent battlefield arms and all that implies by way of soldiers and armies and authoritarianism, then Wu Shu is actually anti-militaristic.

To our way of thinking, an anti-militaristic martial art sounds like nonsense, but this is because we are not Chinese. Chinese culture is rooted in farming and farming communities. A certain amount of collective action to maximise agricultural efficiency is desirable and many large-scale projects such as irrigation, terracing and building benefit from such co-operation. However, while a community is good for farming, a state and all that it implies is not. States are more concerned with territory and boundaries, far less with the practicalities of getting in the crops. The political aspirations of various groups can actively hinder this all-important business.

China suffered a time in her history called the Warring States period. During this time boundaries changed with remarkable frequency. Armies marched and counter-marched, crops were destroyed and ordinary people became highly suspicious of the state, any state, since, from one day to the next, the average peasant family would not know which of these laid claim to their farm. Armies and states became just more pests and threats to the serious business of cultivation. Thus began Wu Shu, the art of stopping the spear, making the aggressive, military behaviour of the state answer to the people.

To this day the Chinese generally prefer to have as little as possible to do with political authority. For many it is axiomatic that the officers of the state are not to be trusted and are to be avoided as much as is humanly possible. This attitude is to be found even in Gong Fusi (Confucius) who lays the duty of disobedience on the people when the ruler is corrupt. This is in spite of his general insistence on preserving the status quo.

MARTIAL ART AND WU SHU

The ideal of Wu Shu is that political, or any other, domination, based upon force of arms, becomes impossible when the individual citizenry are sufficiently skilled to disarm the soldiery. The 'spear' is stopped as a tool of intimidation and manipulation. Now, just in case any reader is running the risk of getting too philosophical, let me emphasise again that none of this thinking derives from anything like our Western liberal traditions. To Chinese folk culture, nothing is as important as getting the harvest in and keeping your family, clan and village going. Communities are useful. States are either irrelevant or pests. In the same way that a farmer ignores the anthill that does no damage to the crop, Chinese peasants preferred to ignore the state. However, when the anthill, or state, becomes a pest then something must be done.

States and armies are very concerned with abstractions like territories, boundaries and obedience. Wu Shu is only concerned with stopping the spear as quickly, neatly and efficiently as possible so that we can then get on with real life. Wu Shu does not care about territory, boundaries or obedience, except when they interfere with cultivation. Thus, Wu Shu allows the people to get on with the important business of living. The harvest has certain rhythms and the water table has its geography. Territories, boundaries and obedience to political authority rarely have anything to do with these.

It is possible for confusion to arise between the martial art of soldiers and the Wu Shu of peasants because the techniques appear similar. There are only a limited number of ways for a human body to move effectively. You can only attempt a certain number of coercive moves, which can then be answered with a number of counter-moves. However, the apparent number of moves can appear to be high because of the number of variations, which can seem almost infinite. There has also been a degree of borrowing and exchange between the martial art of soldier and traditional people's arts, understandably, since most soldiers are recruited from the peasantry and return to their villages if they survive their military careers.

In practice, combative-defensive moves are a bit like cooking. Different cooks will produce meals with different tastes working from the same ingredients. In China there are hundreds, if not thousands, of different systems of Wu Shu. Yet the Masters agree that eventually the differences are more a question of 'flavour', 'taste' or 'style' than anything else. At first students are discouraged from excessive dabbling to reduce confusion and simplify learning. Later, they are encouraged to study more widely to appreciate different systems and realise the commonality that underlies the diversity.

WU SHU, GONG FU AND SELF CULTIVATION

By expanding on the meaning of Wu Shu I hope that I am managing to break down some of the barriers that many people have against studying and practising physical self-defence. I have very little patience with the person who cannot think coherently beyond 'ugh, violence, nasty, bad'. I also hope that I have raised a few questions in the minds of martial artists. I have equally little patience with people whose knee jerk response to certain situations is to jerk it into someone else's guts.

Instead of seeing situations we encounter as 'problems' to be solved, we could see them as 'lessons' to be learned. If we learn our lessons, then those situations are unlikely to trouble us in future. Life is a continually dynamic exercise. No approach is *always correct*. Any approach is sometimes correct. Therefore, an art of self cultivation can be a method of Wu Shu and any method can be used as part of self cultivation.

Here, I shall now briefly cover the meaning of Gong Fu. It has a meaning something like 'regular work' or 'daily exercise'. So, if you were Chinese and watching someone doing their daily routine, you might say that you were watching their 'Gong Fu'. It can also have the meaning of the 'product of regular work' or 'skill', so a cook, a painter, a doctor and a carpenter can all have Gong Fu in their area of specialisation. In South China Gong Fu on its own is understood to be physical Gong Fu, bodily skill. This is most frequently manifested as skill at Wu Shu. From this stems the Western confusion that Gong Fu means 'martial art', since most European contacts with China have come through the south, Canton, Hong Kong and Shanghai.

Taijiquan can be called Gong Fu with just as much legitimacy as other martial art systems such as Wing Chun, Hung Gar, Tong Long or Yi Quan. I once visited a Chinese teacher of Taijiquan and he asked to see my Gong Fu. He might have been asking to see my daily routine, or he might have been asking me to demonstrate my level of skill. Either way, I performed my Taijiquan, which answered his request. I showed him what I do, so he could see how well I could do it.

Self cultivation in any domain can be Gong Fu. In a sense, the Gong Fu of self cultivation is the ultimate Gong Fu – the skill of being yourself, undisturbed by external influences. Any accomplished Qi Gong practitioner will have Gong Fu.

Depending on the particular Qi being worked on, Qi Gong can be self cultivation. You might be practising for a specific purpose, for example to cure a particular ailment. In Chinese medicine the ailment disappears because your Zheng Qi will not support a disordered condition, be it cancer, ulcers, heart disease or infection. Dis-ease is Nature's way of telling you something is wrong. You do not *have a problem* to be solved, rather you are *making a mistake* in the way you are conducting your life. To correct the dis-ease you need to correct the mistake. If your method is the cultivation of your Zheng Qi (essential Qi), then you are cultivating your personal knot of Qi.

TAIJIQUAN AS WU SHU

I hope by now that you have followed the thread from the idea of self cultivation to Qi Gong that underlies Taijiquan. After all, since you are fundamentally Qi, the most direct way to cultivate yourself is to work on your Qi. However, the question still remains as to why Wu Shu is the area for Qi Gong.

Simply put, it is because the context of interpersonal conflict is the one in which most people are likely to find their Qi disrupted. A physical context can also show you most directly how effective your cultivation has been. The Chinese are a very practical people. They have a 'show me' attitude of 'never mind the theory; feel the effect'. All this talk about Qi and waves and energy and Yin and Yang would cut no ice at all, if it did not have demonstrable effects. The Chinese like to test everything. The idea of testing is a very important one in Qi Gong generally and Taijiquan specifically. I shall discuss testing in more detail in the later chapters. For now, it is enough to know that Qi cultivation has to have observable and demonstrable effects.

THREE LEVELS OF TESTING IN TAIJIQUAN

1. *Static testing*: The objective of which is the examination of structure. This is when the Taijiquan player adopts a posture and relaxes into it. This is sometimes called 'holding' a posture but I dislike this expression, since it encourages the use of redundant muscular activity. It is more correct to 'image' the posture and let yourself relax into it. A partner applies pressure to the posture. To the extent that the posture reflects good Qi, both partners will be surprised at the strength that can result from 'doing nothing'.

2. *Moving testing*: The objective now becomes the examination of the success of maintaining structure during movement. The second level of testing requires that a certain amount of success at static testing has been achieved. In this case, the testee moves, according to Qi flow, against a partner's pressure. This helps students to fine-tune their moves. I deliberately use the word pressure, not force or strength, because the tester is not trying to overcome the testee. Many people might be able to do that through strength alone. In moving testing, we use the partner's pressure as a sort of amplifier so that we can find the most efficient and easy movement. Repeated practice of this to enhance the perception of the corrected and refined move dredges the channels so that the Qi flow in the movement is enhanced.

3. *Dynamic testing*: The objective is now the functionality of postures, where it is not a single or simple movement that is being amplified. Dynamic testing requires two people to flow together continuously, without blocking or wasting their Qi. Pushing Hands, Da Lu, and Two Person Taijiquan are, in this sense, dynamic testing. When skilled Taijiquan players step outside the set patterns of these exercises and play spontaneously, this is the highest level of dynamic testing. This is truly stillness in movement. Regardless of what is happening externally, the players are holding to their respective Qi. This requires great skill since, at this level, the interaction can become quite fast. The mind must not become scattered since 'the mind is the commander of the Qi'.

Another way of looking at this ladder of testing is to see it as starting from the mostly physical – static – to the mostly mental – high speed, spontaneous, dynamic. This final level of testing may also be called 'Functional' or 'Application' testing.

THE ROLE OF 'SPARRING' IN TAIJIQUAN

Taijiquan is an art of self cultivation studied by means of the art of stopping the spear. The main aim of self cultivation is a calm, unstressed, peaceful and productive life. The best way to be calm and relaxed is to practise being so in highly stressed conditions. Being attacked is generally regarded as being stressful, which is what studying self cultivation through studying stopping the spear means.

I remember one evening one of my teachers asked me to stay behind after class. It had been a class devoted to the Two Person Taijiquan. I was not particularly surprised, as I had spent quite a lot of time helping my teacher develop his teaching of this aspect of Taijiquan. I provided the human dummy for him to play with. If you are a little slow on the uptake, like me, I can recommend being the dummy for an accomplished Taijiquan player. It is a great way to learn. However, it can be difficult sometimes to be able to talk about what you have learnt in such a direct, physical fashion.

I expected that we would perhaps do some work on moves to be taught in another class. To my surprise, my teacher was in a playful mood and he just said, 'Go on then, hit me.' My first few attempts were a little half hearted, to say the least. But then I got into it and it became faster and freer. I realised then that, to anyone who came in at that point, we would have looked like we were fighting. We were 'fighting' but the fighting was also playing and testing.

This is Taijiquan sparring. It is non-competitive like Aikido but that does not mean that we do not try. If you like, it is a form of 'rough and tumble' play that many other animals enjoy both in youth and maturity. This is playing to improve and to see how well you are doing. For example, at first I thought I was doing well if I could stop my teacher making contact, but later I thought I was getting better if I could make contact with him.

Your opponent is just as much yourself as it is your partner, your weaknesses, failings and slips of concentration. Free sparring is high-level testing to help your self cultivation. Its aim is to be *your* best not *the* best. Trying to be *the* best would mean never losing a fight. This is impossible. Sooner or later we will all lose and it will not matter what excuses you give yourself, like the floor was slippery, I didn't know that technique, my partner was younger/quicker/stronger than me, and so on.

If winning is all that you are interested in and you usually do win or even win all the time, then your interest will eventually fail. Playing to perfect your movement will become boring, and you will give up practice. Without regular exercise, your health will suffer. Should you be so unfortunate as to become involved in a physical confrontation, you will be out of training and may experience very adverse consequences.

A TAIJIQUAN APPROACH TO WU SHU

The art of stopping the spear (Wu Shu) is not really a single art at all. It is the product of the folk cultures of the different regions and peoples of China. Because of this, many different approaches to fighting and ways of dealing with violence can be found within the Wu Shu community, each with particular morals and ethics. In the different schools, these approaches are the strategies and 'fighting theories' particular to each. Taijiquan means something like 'supreme ultimate fist' and this art has great respect from practitioners of other systems.

Since the art exists, and has proven effective, it suggests that there might be alternative ways to understand fighting than in terms of the Roman god Mars. An alternative is the Chinese philosophy of Yin, Yang and Qi. These form the deep foundation of Chinese culture in the same way that ours could be said to have been mainly formed by religious beliefs.

The fantastic shapes that the sea is whipped into during a storm are not 'things' but the result of constructive and destructive interference between different waves – sequences of peaks and troughs. So too, the 'things' of the world can be described as arising from the Qi via Yin and Yang. Spending too much energy focused on the 'thing' approach leads to complexity and diversity of description. It also reinforces and emphasises competition and separateness. Sometimes it results in considering violent escalation as an inevitable result of growth.

Focusing on this 'energetic' and 'oneness' approach emphasises simplicity, unity, co-operation and interdependence. It accepts the variability of intensity as inevitable and sees reversals as essential. While violence is accepted as existing, escalation is seen as controllable.

So what the hell has all this to do with martial art/Wu Shu? It has very little to do with the former but a considerable amount with the latter. Given their approach to everything, the Chinese will expect person-to-person interactions to vary 'energetically'. Of course some interactions will be 'hotter' or 'cooler', more or less intense, high amplitude or low frequency. Since everything is Qi anyway, the peaks and troughs of Yin and Yang are inevitable. Once this variation is accepted, then we can study the art of living. We can learn how to regulate, tame, use or channel these variations. We have to, because we cannot abolish or eliminate them, even if we wanted to.

In human interactions and relationships there is a particular dimension of relevance. We tend to relate to experiences as nice or nasty. We impose value, positive or negative, with varying degrees of intensity. Let's make this more concrete with a few examples.

High positive: Partying, dancing, rough and tumble playing.

High negative: Violence, fighting, rape.

Low positive: Sleeping, relaxing, meditating.

Low negative: Depression, catatonia, anxiety.

We need those things that we value positively. The gut response of nice/nasty has developed because it helped our ancestors to get by, survive and reproduce. However, without the realisation that variation from high to low is inevitable, we can make mistakes. For example, there are people whose fear of violence is so great that they would abolish all high-intensity activity, with the resultant damage that causes. There are also those who fear sloth and burn themselves out by not allowing sufficient time for sleeping, relaxing and meditating.

Taijiquan, as the art of Yin and Yang studied and expressed through the physical discipline of movements of self cultivation applied to the art of stopping the spear, accepts the inevitability of 'violence'. Although this art starts with the study of slow movement, at deeper levels it is important to realise that the complete art goes far beyond this. The same Yin–Yang theory that guides physical self cultivation can also be applied as a life strategy or 'fighting theory'.

We cannot exist in totally unchanging conditions. We, like everything else, are dynamic and need occasional high-energy activities. If this need is not recognised, some people go out to create such interactions. Tai Chi philosophy says that there is always a Yin and a Yang. Every Yin has Yang within, every Yang has Yin. Thus, there is a Yin way and a Yang way to deal with situations. The Taiji way is not to get stuck in either Yin or Yang.

Encountering a high-energy situation, a 'violent' encounter, the Yin option is to try and change the value of the situation from negative to positive. The energy in the situation is not what makes the situation 'violent', it is the value attached to the energy that makes it 'violent'. Some people are so inexperienced in energy management that they will automatically attach a negative value and label any energy level, above what they feel comfortable with, as 'violent'. Having made this decision and fixed the value, then the situation is 'violent'. They have cut themselves off from any other options.

Yin gives birth to Yang. Therefore, when the Yin option is not available, there can only be Yang. At this level, Yang is the energy management option and this can be implemented with a higher or lower level of skill. People without experience, practice or training can expect to manage the energy poorly and this may result in damage to themselves. This damage may be physical or psychological. People who have been mugged, even when they have not suffered physically, can be deeply upset by the eruption of 'violence' into their otherwise placid lives. Their inexperience prevents them from channelling the energy into personally useful, or at least minimally harmful, damage limitation.

So here we have a sort of paradox. People with experience of the Yang solution are better able to apply the Yin solution. If you have experience of high-energy physical interactions, you do not have to jump to the conclusion that a particular situation is negative. You have room to manoeuvre before deciding that you are involved in a 'violent' encounter. Then there is another paradox. Having decided that this is a 'violent' encounter, the trained, or experienced, person can channel the energy and perhaps reduce the damage to a minimum. What this minimum might be in any particular situation can vary enormously. Taking the most extreme case, a minimum might need the death of one, or even more, people. We must never ignore or hide from this possibility. Hesitation might mean that you are the dead person. Taking another life is always very serious.

A less extreme 'damage minimum' might be that of so many Gong Fu myths, or pieces of 'wild history'. When attacked, the Master preaches a sermon on the virtues of a harmonious, non-violent, approach to life – using hands, fists and feet. The former assailant is spiritually enlightened on the spot and becomes a devoted disciple. As an ideal, that is a nice myth to aspire to. More realistically, we could summarise this as having to defend yourself physically and succeeding.

Sometimes 'damage limitation' might mean giving in to the 'violence', or perhaps I should say, appearing to give in. If a group of armed individuals want your wallet, I'd say, 'Let them have it.' What is the point of surrendering your life of self cultivation, endlessly interesting and fruitful as it is, just for a wallet? There are many scenarios in which the most effective use of your skills is not to use them. You might lose your wallet but, when you make it *your* choice, you will minimise the damage to your self-image that some people suffer after such an incident.

A PERSONAL ENCOUNTER

This is all very abstract and perhaps difficult to really get to grips with, so I'll tell you a story from my own experience. The fact that I am the focus of this story is irrelevant. Some time ago, I went for a drink with two friends, a man and a woman. Because the woman had been the victim of rape, she was in the habit of carrying a knife in her handbag, which helped her to feel more 'secure'. I very definitely do not approve of this idea. First it is illegal, a concealed weapon, so its possession alone, carried for 'self-defence' or not, increases the chance of hassle in your life. Who needs extra interference from the officers of the state? Second, tools that you do not know how to control have a tendency to result in damage to the owner.

After the pub closed the three of us said goodbye to our friends and set off to catch the train home. By the time we got to the station, my male friend and I needed to offload some of the beer we had drunk. We were catching the last train and the station was fairly quiet. My woman friend said that she would wait for us, as she did not need the loo, having sensibly availed herself of the pub's facilities.

Off we went, with me finishing as quickly as possible so as not to leave my friend unaccompanied too long. By the time I returned, alone, I could see that she was talking to three young men. One of them had his arm around her waist. As I came closer, I could see that the young men were somewhat the worse for wear. I also realised that they had probably been to a football match as they were wearing team coloured scarves and woolly hats. They were trying to solicit my friend with what my granny would have called 'improper suggestions'. Needless to say, she did not look very happy.

None of them had seen my approach and I was very concerned about the knife in the handbag. I definitely did not want that to come out and further complicate the situation, so to control the knife was my first priority. I walked up gently and locked the wrist and arm of the man with his arm round my friend's waist. Using the stiff arm as a lever, I threw him about eight feet away. I did not throw him to the floor. I did not use any pain against his joints. I had an option to break his elbow. I chose not to do this. I simply shoved him away. He had been on her left as he disappeared, to be replaced by me on her right. I put my arm round her waist, partly to reassure her, and partly to get my arm over her handbag to keep it shut. I then used peripheral vision to check where that man was and started talking football to his two mates.

Now, I'm not very interested in football and I don't know very much about it. But they were drunk enough to be slow and easily confused and I don't believe that they were very sure what had happened. Suddenly, it must have seemed to them, the 'spare' woman was not 'spare' or 'fair game' anymore. By talking about the game they had been to watch – their team had lost – I changed the situation. When their mate reappeared, he too was a little confused. However, since everyone was chatting in a friendly fashion and my male friend then arrived back from the loo, the potential situation completely collapsed. We commiserated with them for their loss and then went our separate ways as our respective trains came in.

Looking back they seemed nice enough blokes. They were just looking for something to cheer themselves up. They had had a drink or two and were looking for female company. The fact that their strategy was hardly likely to impress my female friend did not seem to have dawned on them. There are thousands of men, old and young, who have such attitudes to a woman apparently alone. She is 'obviously fair game'. Since this is a book about Taijiquan, I will say no more than that I find such attitudes a pathetic apology for any genuine form of masculinity.

The general principle of Tai Chi fighting strategy is to encourage smoothness of energy flow. A favourite metaphor is the round of the seasons. Any given day might be stormy, or hot, or exhibit any intensity of energy, but the seasons flow on smoothly, despite this local, or individual, variation. The individual variation might be unpredictable or uncontrollable but the overall trend is smooth.

Society is like the round of the year; it is the sum of the individuals and individual interactions, which are like the days of the year. Variability for individuals and days is needed as a source of growth. Mostly this variability at the individual level cancels out and the big circles smoothly carry on. If harmony is not cared for, or variability is over-controlled, then trends can combine and interact to disrupt the greater flow. Global warming is a good example of such disruption. War can also be seen as a particular outcome of combining and interacting trends. The individual variations are chained together to create what might be called 'social' warming. The energy flow becomes too intense and harsh.

This is the Taiji understanding of the need for Wu Shu. When the people are skilled in self cultivation via Wu Shu, this helps to regulate or 'police' society. A common Taijiquan Wu Shu goal is to be a military police officer, which is someone who can police the military. The ideal is that, if everyone knew and shared this philosophy and accompanying skills, the military would become redundant. At the same time, what external aggressor could impose their will on such a community? Entering this community's territory might be easy, but possessing it would be very difficult, if not impossible. Very soon the invader would be either absorbed or give up and leave such a land of ungovernable people. The history of China shows the success of this strategy.

CONCLUSION

I have taken a lot of words to explain my understanding of the vexed question of Taijiquan as a 'martial art'. I expect that I may have annoyed many people but I do not wish anyone to feel that I am criticising their practice. The community of Taijiquan players is very large and each player's practice will vary according to preference, capacity and opportunity. My only concern is for the art, and that it will be passed on to future generations as completely as it was handed down from the past. Any individual's practice is a personal matter. We all take what we need and what we can digest. We all grow in the art at our own rates. For some, the higher levels of practice may not be possible, but I feel passionately that this art of Taijiquan is more than my personal practice and understanding, or yours, or anyone else's. It hurts me to see dissension among my brothers and sisters in Taijiquan and I fear that this may damage the passage of the art to our successors.

Finally I will close with a quote from Yang Cheng Fu:

Learning self-defence applications is indispensable in Taijiquan. Students who are primarily interested in exercise must also study applications. If they don't, it becomes very dull and the majority will quit. In fact, ignoring the applications is also an obstacle to making progress in strengthening the body.

The purpose of mastering self-defence applications is not to bully people, but to study the marvellous principles with friends. You attack and I neutralise; I attack and you respond. It flows on and on without end. Every kind of change can take place without exhausting the possibilities. If one realises that there are infinite variations in Taijiquan, with dancing hands and stepping feet, then the interest increases daily. With practice over the years, this continuous and unforgettable joy greatly strengthens the body. To train the body it is important to study the applications and even more so if one expects to face opponents. Therefore friends, when practising Taijiquan, it is absolutely necessary to study the applications. (Wile 1983, p.149)

Part II

Initial Foundation

Chapter 4

Returning to Nature: Restoring Spring

The previous chapters have discussed the 'what' of Taijiquan. It is now time for us to turn our attention to the 'how' of this art. There is a syllabus for learning Taijiquan but, because it is a holistic art, the journey through its various facets is not a simple, direct progression. The later or more advanced levels of practice feed back to both develop and refine our understanding and practice of the basics.

Writing this book is a top-down approach to Taijiquan. I have started with the most general and abstract ideas of Chinese culture to try and explain the nature of the exercise. I believe that this approach is necessary because we, as Western students, do not have the advantage of absorbing basic Chinese ideas in childhood.

The traditional way of teaching is bottom up. The teacher gives very little background or theoretical information. Students are simply told, 'Do this. Put your feet here…your hands there.' Students are often expected to work out for themselves why a move is done in a certain way, or why a teacher says that something is wrong. The student who fails to grasp the teacher's point in two or three repetitions will usually be left to their own devices.

This method is not really appropriate for Western students. We are less able to develop our experiences in class because we are not part of the living traditions of Chinese culture. We often cannot comprehend the teacher's throw-away remarks or references to popular and classical literature. Furthermore, our culture teaches us to expect to be given the context for learning almost anything. We have been trained to need to know 'why'. So, in addition to telling you 'how' to follow the way of Taijiquan, I have to tell you 'what' the way of Taijiquan is, and 'why' it is that way.

THE MEANING OF NATURAL IN TAIJIQUAN

I have said before that there is a syllabus for Taijiquan, despite the absence of a grading system. Where does this syllabus come from? The Chinese might say that it comes from the Tao, the Natural Way. So, what is this Tao, or, more specifically, what is it in relation to the art of Taijiquan?

The standard or set of standards that we use as our yardstick are provided by the 'Laws of Heaven and Earth' themselves; that is, Tao, the Way of Nature, or Natural Way. This brings us to a very important point concerning the use of the word 'natural'. We use this word in two distinct ways that can be in some conflict with each other.

First, we use 'natural' to mean according to nature. In the West, we might say according to the 'laws of science' as they apply to people specifically, which implies according to physics, anatomy, biomechanics, physiology and so forth. In China, of course, 'natural' means in accord or harmony with the Laws of Heaven and Earth, following the Tao as it applies to people.

The other use of the word 'natural' is something like frequent, familiar or usual. To a heavy coffee drinker, six to eight cups a day is 'natural'. To a coal miner, working narrow seams, it might be 'natural' to spend much of the working day hunched over and straining. However, both of these seem poor examples of according with the Laws of Heaven and Earth.

The application of the Laws of Heaven and Earth to our bodies allows us to cultivate our selves in a Natural fashion. Our habitual ways of being may be 'natural' to us as individuals, but whether they are natural for human beings, or indeed any living things, cannot be taken for granted. I call this first stage, or task, the Rectification of the body.

THE RECTIFICATION OF THE BODY

This is a term I have borrowed from the neo-Confucians. The idea of Rectification comes from the continuity of Chinese history and the veneration of the ancestors. The Chinese view is that the ancestors said all that was needed about life, the universe and everything. However, they recognise that the world changes and develops, 'grows'. The ancestors may have grasped the knot of life, but while we unravel this knowledge, the understanding will also need to grow, thus leading to the need for 'Rectification' from time to time.

As understanding and knowledge grow, so there is a need to keep re-expressing the ancestors' wisdom in ways that are fruitful, comprehensible and useful to today's generation. Lao Nai-hsuan, Richard Wilhelm's collaborator in his famous translation of the *I Ching*, put it this way:

> In the words and deeds of the past there lies a hidden treasure that men may use to strengthen and elevate their own characters. The way to study the past is not to confine oneself to

mere knowledge of history but, through application of this knowledge, to give actuality to the past. (Baynes 1977)

I feel that this is as good a way as any to describe the fruitful study and practice of Taijiquan itself.

The need for Rectification, either occasionally or regularly, is hardly surprising. Life can be a demanding experience with various ups and downs, knocks and bumps. Merely keeping going causes a certain amount of wear and tear. However, we are, frankly, naive about our bodies and their use and capabilities. We all tend to passively accept the creeping degeneration that we call 'getting old', yet we are fully aware, in our machine age, that regular maintenance and occasional adjustment are essential to ensure long, trouble-free running and use. A car that is not properly serviced on a regular basis has a 'life' that is just a fraction of one properly cared for. If this is true for 'hard' machines like trains, boats, cars and planes, then how much more likely is it to be true of 'soft' machines like people and other animals? How much of the gradual loss of function that we accept as part of ageing could be due to lack of maintenance?

Some people will point to the wonderful self-repair and maintenance capacity of the 'soft' machine and claim that that is all there is to it. This is fatalistic in the extreme. It ranks with the arguments against the train – if God had meant people to go that fast, we would have been given wheels – and against the plane – we would have been given wings – with similar arguments against anything from aqualungs to zeppelins. Some people claim that it is anti-human, anti-evolutionary, anti-life and even blasphemous to try to know better than God how the divine and creative gifts that are part of the Laws of Heaven and Earth should unfold. Many would also say that these are particular and unique in people.

What is 'natural' for us as individuals, groups, cultures or societies may not be 'natural' in the sense of conforming to the Laws of Heaven and Earth. In fact, what we consider to be 'natural' to us is merely familiar and is anything but an expression of our inner nature. Certain 'natural' postures, ways of moving and using our bodies can owe more to fashion and social pressure than to nature or the Tao. What we consider 'natural' movement may, in fact, be disadvantageous. It may be life depleting rather than life enhancing, possibly even damaging or fatal, in the long term.

THE NEED FOR A TEACHER

This is where the wonderful flexibility, adaptability and learning capacity that we possess as human beings can betray us. This is why the Chinese emphasise the need for a teacher, especially in the initial stages of learning. It is all very well being told that Taiji or Qi Gong is 'natural' and 'easy'. However, for many beginners, certainly for myself in my own early days, the moves, gestures, postures and rules seem anything but 'natural'. I felt clumsy and awkward, while the work was definitely work, and not very noticeably 'easy'. At first, a teacher is very necessary to point out deviations from natural in the sense of in harmony with the Tao and also to help us avoid degenerating into the crude 'natural' of just familiar.

This is also where the interpretation of the classical verse 'First in the mind and then in the body' becomes important. It is essential that understanding precedes action, particularly for people who have not grown up with Chinese culture. Understanding is necessary to substitute for the internalisation of the concepts of Tao and harmony with nature. Without understanding, many of the forms of Qi Gong, especially soft styles and Taiji in particular, can all too easily degenerate into exercises that preserve poor functional habits.

When I first started Taijiquan, I naively thought that it was impossible to do it so badly as to damage health. Sadly, I now realise that this is not true. People do seem to have a great capacity to misuse almost everything. From my observations, some students, due to a combination of poor practice and limited understanding, develop impaired functions after a few years. This reflects the two Chinese proverbs: 'There are no bad students, only bad teachers', and 'Qi Gong is easy to learn and hard to correct'.

THE RECTIFIED BODY

With that entire preamble out of the way, we can now turn to a description of a 'Rectified' body. The discussion, so far, may have seemed rather vague and philosophical, using words and phrases like the Laws of Heaven and Earth, harmony, Tao and Natural. I hope that this has begun to make a certain kind of sense. However, now we find the delightful practicality of the Chinese coming into play. The bottom line for the Chinese is 'Does it work? Does it make a difference?' In the long term the suggestion underlying all these ideas is that, by being in harmony, we will ensure a life of maximum quality and quantity. However, who wants to wait twenty, thirty, forty or more years to find out if you've had an extended life? Could there be other yardsticks that we can use in the shorter term? Otherwise all our exercise and effort could be empty and ineffective or, as the Chinese would say, 'Flower fist and brocade leg'.

We must begin to bring all this down to the practicalities of day to day living. Information must make a difference or it is not information at all, just pretty words. The central idea that we need to grasp, in order to make all these ideas workable, is the concept Qi, which has already been discussed at length. Let us just recap what we mean by Qi. Qi is the essence of living as opposed to non-living things. It is pattern, flow, organisation and movement. It is the coherent, organising tendency that creates and sustains life. Intimately associated with breathing, it is not breath alone. Present in movement, it is not movement itself. For those of you with an understanding of radio waves, it seems to be both the carrier wave and the information carried by the wave.

An abundance of Qi is a prerequisite for robust health, with a deficiency of Qi leading to ill health or disease. What we in the West see as the symptoms of specific ailments are, to a traditional Chinese doctor, only the secondary consequences of trouble with Qi and its circulation. Their main aim is to restore the Qi circulation. The ailment itself is not ignored but, without rebalancing the Qi, a full recovery is held to be unlikely. Once again using the radio wave analogy, rebalancing the Qi is something like 'cleaning up' or 'reducing the noise' in the signal. Pursuing this analogy a little, health can be seen as a high ratio of signal over noise. As noise increases, the organisation of the information in the signal declines. Finally, if noise triumphs there is no information left and the result of that information – in this case a particular knot of Qi: an individual life – disappears.

THE RECTIFIED BODY: NO BLOCKING OR WASTING

Equipped with the idea of Qi, we are now ready to discuss the means to Rectify the body. The simple traditional prescription is 'No blocking, no wasting'. In Rectification the Qi is often described as being like a fluid or liquid but this does not mean that it is so. In a similar way, the flow of electricity is often explained with reference to a fluid model.

The liquid or fluid model is used to explain the flowing and circulating nature of Qi. The Chinese have been familiar with water engineering, particularly agricultural irrigation, for a very long time. It is natural that they should use the technology that they are most comfortable with to model Qi effects. We have done much the same in the West. In particular, psychological theories have a history of reflecting contemporary technologies. Freud's theories have a hydraulic or steam engineering framework, then for a while it was fashionable to talk about the brain as a giant telephone switchboard. Currently computer models are fashionable.

A comparison with irrigation ditches can be used to demonstrate the two key ideas of 'blocking' and 'wasting'. Rubbish falling into a ditch will restrict the movement of the water. Similarly, the flow of Qi is restricted when the channels along which it passes are blocked. In the body, Qi generally gets blocked at joints when they are incorrectly positioned or aligned.

Continuing this comparison, if the water in the ditch overflows and floods the wrong field, it is being wasted. The

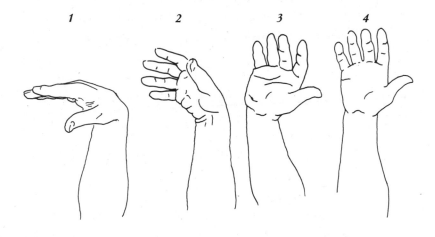

Blocking at the wrist. 1–3 blocked; 4 correct

'wasting' of Qi generally arises when there is excessive tension in the muscles. Excessive tension reveals itself in two ways. The first is when unnecessary muscles are working. If, when you hold your arm out horizontal, parallel to the floor, you find that your bicep is hard, you will be wasting Qi as it is completely unnecessary to use this muscle to hold your arm out.

The second is the development of fatigue. When the amount of tension in a given muscle is not varying smoothly, following the changes in the load on it, that tension is greater than necessary. This means that it becomes fatigued more quickly. When it is fatigued, its ability to respond smoothly to changes becomes jerky. This then leads to various over and under shoots, which are themselves fatiguing.

From the injunction 'no blocking', we come to understand that posture, structure and alignment are important, especially their preservation in movement. From 'no wasting', we develop the idea that relaxation is important. This has two facets. Physically, we can expect that muscular tensions should be kept to the minimum. However, mental relaxation is of equal importance, as we all know that mental and physical tension can be connected, e.g. the classic 'tension' headache.

In the West, our enthusiasm and our determination to succeed often makes us try too hard, physically and mentally. We have generally been brought up to value effort and hard work. We frown, tense and grit our teeth, grunt and vocalise to demonstrate our level of effort.

Much of this performance, often sub-conscious, is aimed at others, initially parents, family and teachers, later employers and work mates. It is not directed towards the task in hand. So what else can we call it but wasted energy (wasted Qi)?

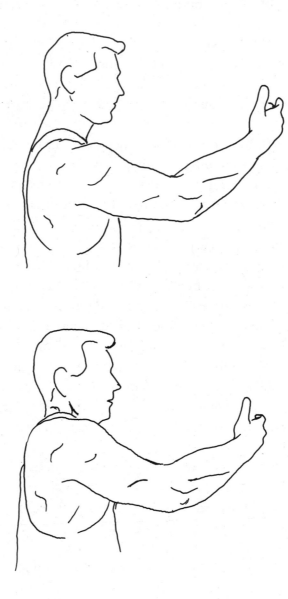

Blocking and wasting in the arm: Upper correct; Lower both blocked and wasted

NATURAL ALIGNMENT

We obviously want to be able to make the task of Rectification something real and 'do-able'. This means we must have a clear idea of the necessary actions to take. So now we could do with a clearer idea of what is meant by alignment. Where can we find a source of ideas to develop the aspect of 'no blocking' further? Since our yardstick is the Laws of Heaven and Earth, where else is there to look but in the natural world all around us? In particular, we need to look at the domain of four-limbed living things, since we clearly belong to this pattern. But first let us notice that we are unique in our vertical, two-legged way of standing and moving. This then becomes our first and most important axis of alignment, so no blocking or wasting along this axis is our first goal.

If we needed any further reason to accept the importance of this vertical axis, we have only to remember how common back problems are. Not blocking the spine is usually expressed in Qi Gong as 'hanging from the top of the head'. More accurately, this is saying that the spine needs to be gently stretched both upwards and downwards. I sometimes think of this as a type of self-traction. It is most easily achieved by visualising the head as being suspended from above. In the classical writings of Taijiquan, we find such phrases as 'pigtail tied to the rafters', 'head floating on the neck' or 'the energy at the top of the head should be light and sensitive'. A good little trick, especially indoors, is to feel that your nose is nearer to the roof than the floor. At the same time, imagining that you have a weight attached to the tip of your coccyx triggers the downward lengthening. Many people unconsciously lift their coccyx. Technically the 'Wei Lu' point (located on the tip of the final coccygeal vertebra) must be vertical.

Hanging in the gravity field and gently extending the spine helps to reduce blocking on the uniquely human

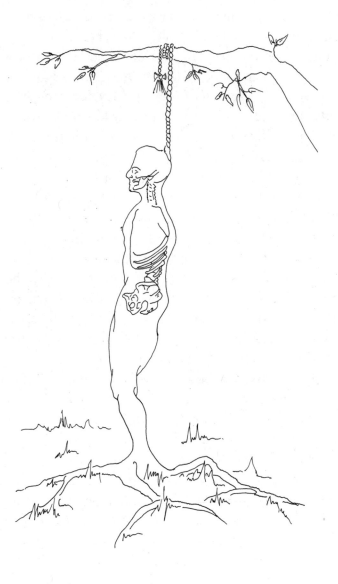

Extending the spine

vertical axis. But what about wasting? In common with all other four-limbed animals, people are three-dimensional. We now have an idea about one of the major axes of the body, so let us look at another one.

The muscles on either side of the spine are areas where Qi might be wasted. The vertical axis along the spine can be viewed like a hinge or the spine of a book where the left and right sides of the body are the two covers. The question arises, what is the 'natural' angle between the two sides? Should the two sides be folded back making the chest prominent, or should they be folded forwards, making the back fuller and more expanded?

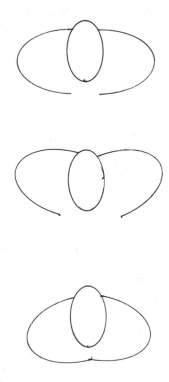

Chest blocking: Upper correct; Middle too open; Lower too closed

STRUCTURE AND POSTURE

Where can we look to find the answer? In the West we have received plenty of advice about posture, chest out, shoulders back, stomach in – as my aunt in the Women's Royal Air Force (WRAF) used to insist. We have such an obsession with the chest – out, projected – and the stomach – flat – and the legs – long – that we even have high-heeled shoes, elevating us, and tending to force the chest out, the stomach in and emphasising long-legged postures.

We now know that high-heeled shoes are bad for the back, not to mention encouraging corns, bunions and a tendency to fall. It seems likely that, even without the heels, this postural prescription is a long way from being natural or in harmony with the Laws of Heaven and Earth. It seems to owe more to fashion, ritual and posturing than to physics, anatomy or biomechanics.

THE APPLICATION OF YIN–YANG TO THE BODY

By contrast the Taoist biologists and doctors in China have always acknowledged the continuum that connects people with all other living things, especially four-limbed creatures. From their observations of the general features of the four-limbed pattern, they developed certain principles. Perhaps the most important of these was the application of Yin–Yang analytical theory.

Yin–Yang theory is the foundation of Chinese science. It is a theory that permits generalised observations to be made and has a similar role to that of algebra in Western science. It is a more qualitative, analytical framework than the quantitative base of algebra, but there are similarities. Just as algebra permits the development of general equations of motion that are applicable to the motion of any moving body, Yin–Yang theory develops general expressions of relationship.

The first application of Yin–Yang theory to four-limbed animals is deciding which surfaces of the body are Yin and which are Yang. This is the nature of Yin–Yang analysis. It is hierarchical, dividing into Yin and Yang and then repeating the division, since any Yin or Yang can always be divided further into another Yin–Yang pair.

The most common four-limbed pattern is to have limbs of more or less equal length with a four-legged gait. Primates, including us, are clearly modifications of the basic 'leg at each corner' design. Two major principles emerge from this observation.

First is the none too obvious conclusion that the back of the torso is Yang and the front is Yin. A four-legged animal can be viewed as consisting of its structure and the space it naturally encloses.

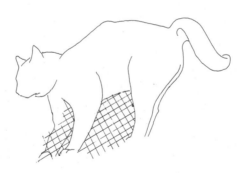

Cat Yin–Yang showing contained volume

That space can be regarded, in a certain sense, as part of the animal because the four-legged stance and gait consistently encloses a slightly variable volume. Yin–Yang theory defines inner surfaces as Yin and outer surfaces as Yang. Yin is concave and Yang convex; Yin is space and Yang content. In the language of Western biology, the dorsal surface is Yang and the ventral Yin.

The second principle is that breathing is abdominal. The spine and four limbs, one at each corner, function similarly to a ridge tent with two 'A' frames, one at each end.

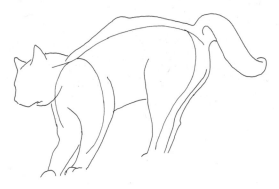

Cat 'A' frame

To grasp this point, think about four-legged animals and their breathing patterns. Look at a cat, dog or horse. They all breathe abdominally. They have to, as their four-legged stance and gait will not permit anything else. If you can't observe animals, you can bend down and see how you breathe in a posture with all four limbs on the ground. If you try this, be cautious, since we are no longer capable of four-legged motion and this posture is a little strenuous, particularly on the neck. This helps us to understand some of the verses found in the Taijiquan classics, for example 'Strength is stored in the spine, and issued from the back', and 'Sink the chest and raise the back'. The latter verse is particularly prone to misunderstanding. Among the many benefits that flow from the understanding of this verse comes an improved use of the lungs. It eventually will help us to understand the emphasis on the lower Dantien (one of three spheres of the 'organ' Sanjiao that sits within the pelvis), abdominal breathing and the Taijiquan emphasis of 'Elbow to Knee'. The Wuji point identified by Qi Gong practitioners is located at the centre of the sphere of the lower Dantien: it is when the internal vertical line, called the Zhong Mai, produced when the acupoint Bai Hui (on the crown of the head) is vertically aligned with the acupoint Hui Yin (on the floor of the pelvis), is bisected, at an angle of 90 degrees, by the horizontal line between the Ming Men acupoint (of the Du Mai meridian on the spine) and the acupoint Qi Hai (of the Ren Mai meridian approximately two inches below the navel). The lower Dantien is illustrated in the figure on p.181.

However, moving on from the breathing of four-legged animals, we also come to the question of how to breathe when physically or emotionally stressed. We tend to heave our breastbones up and down after exertion, or when emotionally stressed. Four-legged animals cannot breathe this way without falling down. When they need to breathe more deeply, the breath expands up from the abdomen, causing the flanks to heave due to the movement of the ribs. You can also try this in your 'four-legged' position to feel it work. Alternatively, press both hands onto your breastbone and take a series of deep breaths.

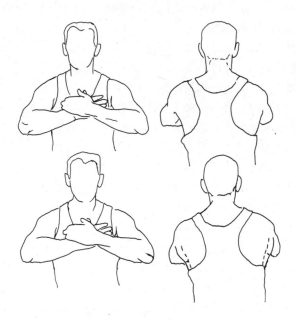

Breathing into the flanks, NB lower back view

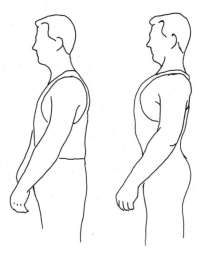

Raising the chest blocks the spine

Your hands will prevent the breastbone from moving, and you will find that your ribs will expand forwards and round from your spine. This is the meaning of 'Sink the chest'. It will also make the emphasis on breathing from the lower Dantien understandable.

Because we are three-dimensional, it is impossible to lift the breastbone without having an effect on the spine. If the bottom of the breastbone lifts, it must pull the spine inwards, which blocks the spine and puts a distinct kink into the major vertical axis, the lower back. This is a particular problem with our human variant of the basic four-limbed pattern.

This consideration of structure answers the questions about how the rest of the body should relate to the vertical axis, and gives us an

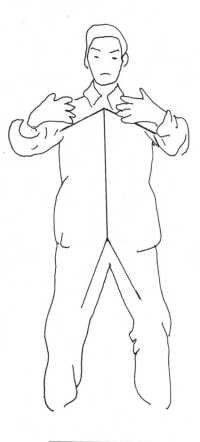

Vertical human 'A' frame

insight into breathing. The Western view of 'chest out, stomach in, shoulders back' is completely back to front. It strives to make the Yin into Yang, and the Yang into Yin, by inflating and projecting the chest while hollowing the back and depressing the spine. It is revealed as just show, or a 'front'. Not surprisingly, this is bad for our overall maintenance, not least because it inhibits breathing efficiency.

In summary, given the importance of the vertical axis, the spine should be like the ridgepole of a double 'A' frame tent, with the upper arms to the elbows one 'A' frame and the thighs to the knees the other. Obviously, due to our vertical stance, the model of the ridgepole and 'A' frames has to be stood on one 'A' frame.

We are now getting somewhere in our quest to discover how to 'Rectify' the body in conformity with the Laws of Heaven and Earth. However, we still have some way to go in order to define a complete set of principles to cover the whole body in all three dimensions.

We have been deciphering the meaning of several classical verses and proverbs, but how do we interpret the rest? For example, 'The whole body should be round'; what could this mean? We also have an unanswered question about relaxation. Having realised that there is a connection between not wasting Qi and being relaxed, how relaxed is relaxed? Relax too much and we will just collapse in a heap on the floor. These questions will be the subject of the following chapters.

CONCLUSION

In this chapter we have begun to discover the syllabus of Taijiquan. Unlike other systems, Taijiquan is not simply a collection of techniques, but is also organic and developmental. Taijiquan grows rather than being assembled. The syllabus of Taijiquan is better viewed as the attainment of developmental stages rather than as the mechanical learning of techniques. As an animal develops from infancy, through childhood, to adolescence and finally adulthood so do we, in our Taijiquan practice. There is a proverb from the old schools: 'First we crawl. Then we walk. Then we run. Perhaps with persistence some may even learn to fly.'

The first developmental task is to return the body to a more Natural condition. What Natural means comes from a study of the natural world of living things through Yin–Yang analysis. Traditionally, this is called removing blockages and preventing wasting of Qi. I have borrowed from the neo-Confucians by calling this the 'Rectification of the body'.

There are many techniques that can be used at this stage. Standing and relaxing into specific postures is often helpful. For people who find this difficult or stressful, slow considered movement such as Taijiquan forms are an alternative. They should be performed very softly, using the imagination to picture, and feel oneself hanging like a puppet. The use of both methods together can speed up progress. The objective is to achieve the 'A' frame structure within all your postures.

What an unskilled person sees is limited, since they do not know what to look for. A Master, or teacher, will be able to know if a student needs to work on returning to nature, or is at a more advanced stage. It should be said that it is not worth trying to increase your Qi without first making sure that your body is clear enough to take it. As one of my teachers put it, 'Before increasing the pressure in the pipes we must make sure that the plumbing is OK.'

Chapter 5

Learning How to Learn

In the last chapter, we began our detailed study of the 'how' of Taijiquan, which I call 'Rectification' of the body. The traditional description is 'No blocking, no wasting' or sometimes 'Returning to nature'. However, just having an idea about correct structure is not enough. Clearing your structure can result in achieving a condition of 'No blocking' and may give a superficial appearance of Rectification, or returning to nature. However, if the other half of the traditional prescription is not also followed, you will not succeed. 'No wasting' is just as important.

DON'T TRY TOO HARD

I hope you will have understood that a Natural body should follow the four-limbed pattern common to all four-legged animals. The major and unique difference, for humans, is the fact that we stand upright on our two hind limbs. Nevertheless, we are still Yin on the inside, and Yang on the outside, hence all the classical advice about the spine, chest and abdominal breathing. For Westerners, who tend to try too hard, being shown the Natural structure might actually make things worse. When we try too hard to achieve this posture, we will inevitably waste Qi and so fail. If Qi is being wasted, then the posture cannot be called natural. Nevertheless, many of us will be tempted to try and get a Natural posture. This arises from a misunderstanding of the word 'should'. People often use the word 'should' when they are uncomfortable about saying 'must'. This happens so often that, by the time we are adult, most of us understand 'should' as a command.

SHOULD IS A CONDITION – NOT A COMMAND

Parents and teachers often tell children that they 'should' be polite and well behaved. Breaking this rule leads to admonition so they grow up understanding 'should' to mean 'must'. As adults this fiction is maintained. We are told that we 'should' turn up to work on time. No, we *must* turn up to work on time. That is the nature of most employment contracts. This confusion between 'should' and 'must' causes a great deal of human suffering. Happiness is occasionally considered to be a Natural condition. We think we should be happy. But, if you think that 'should' means 'must', then you will try to be happy instead of examining your circumstances, or behaviour, to discover what is being missed. So, on top of the original discomfort, you add the task of trying to achieve something, in this case the happiness that would, in fact, naturally arise in the absence of the sources of discomfort.

WEI WU-WEI

'Wei Wu-Wei' means to become more aware of, and then work on improving, our automatic processes. When I say that a 'Rectified' or 'Natural' body should have a certain structure, it is vital that you do not think that I am giving a set of instructions. I don't want you to think that my description of the non-blocked structure is in any way like my WRAF auntie's commands: 'Chest out, shoulders back, stomach in.'

I hope you will understand that increasing success at not blocking your Qi will lead your structure to grow more and more like my description. You will be able to measure how well you are doing by the extent to which it matches this description. Remember, I am describing your target, I am not telling you that you 'must' hold yourself this way.

I can hear you asking, 'How can we practise at all if you are telling us not to try to get a Rectified, Natural body? Is there anything we can do?' Yes, there is, but it will be a very different kind of doing than what you might expect. In Chinese it is called Wei Wu-Wei. 'Wei' means to do, to make things, to be self-conscious of your actions. It is a uniquely human verb. People do (Wei) things all the time. I'm writing this book, we build houses, roads, barns, spaceships and kidney dialysis machines.

'Wu' is a negative participle and it has no equivalent in European languages. It belongs to a group of sounds that are not words as such, but markers that tell you something about the words in a sentence. We might consider them as audible punctuation. Mandarin Chinese needs these markers because it is a tonal language. In spoken English a question can be inferred by the tone of my voice. Sometimes this can be sarcastic and you will realise that I mean the opposite of what has been said. Written English can use the verb pronoun inversion, e.g. 'Are you going to the shops?', but in everyday conversation I'm more likely to say 'You're going to the shops' and raise my tone as I get to the end of the sentence. In writing the same structure can be used but with a question mark at the end: 'You're going to the shops?' When you read the sentence with a question mark, you can 'hear' the rising tone inside your head.

Since, in Mandarin, the tone is part of the word, the Chinese need the equivalent of verbal punctuation marks. The sound 'Ma' with the correct tone is a question. With different tones it also means 'mother', or 'horse', so you can see why getting the tone right is important. Similarly, 'Wu' in 'Wu-Wei' means that whatever comes next is to be understood as negative or opposite. It is most frequently translated as 'not doing', which is not incorrect, but is not very helpful either.

The Chinese natural scientists use Wu-Wei in a very particular, technical way. They observed that there is always a lot going on in nature. All living things are 'doing' something all the time. As you read this, you are digesting, breathing; your heart is beating and so on. If there are plants, animals or insects near you, they are all 'doing' their vital processes too.

However, this type of Natural 'doing' is different from the purely human 'doing' of 'Wei', the self-conscious action. It is a kind of doing that just happens, without conscious volition. We can 'do' our breathing and even 'do' not-breathing. However, if we do not breathe, we will pass out and breathing will start up again. This is a very good example of Wu-Wei. Therefore, Wu-Wei means that kind of doing that is not like the self-conscious kind. Sometimes it is translated as 'growing', so we could say that babies, young animals and plants Wu-Wei from immaturity to maturity.

The way to practise self cultivation is 'Wei Wu-Wei', which means 'doing not-doing'. One of my students explained his Taijiquan practice by saying, 'In class we practise spontaneous actions (not-doing) so that in life, when we need to be spontaneous, we can act spontaneously (not-doing) properly.' This illustrates the 'bottom-up' nature of the traditional relationship between the Taiji teachers and their students. It also illustrates how, traditionally, students are passive and do exactly what they are told. Returning to nature is not something they 'do', rather it is something they find, or discover or re-learn, with the help of their teacher. At first, we may be so blind and deaf to our Natural 'not-doing' that we need to surrender 'doing' to the teacher. At least in the beginning, we have to let the teacher tell us how to move and where to put our arms and legs. Because teachers have an internal and external knowledge of 'No blocking, no wasting', we can trust their advice. Teachers do not teach Taiji, or Taijiquan, they help, or make, us learn what our bodies are made to do naturally. In a way it can be compared to sculpture: we just 'take away' everything that isn't a cat, or an eagle, or whatever the sculptor is creating.

There is a sense in which, however distorted our body might have become, with Qi blocked and wasted all over the place, this is nevertheless still Natural. It is the Natural result of the 'doing' and 'not-doing' that has brought us to this moment. The art of self cultivation is to bring your 'doing' to the support of your 'not-doing'. This unifies your self and so empowers your being. Wei Wu-Wei is probably one of the most important and practical instructions I can give.

I am sure that you will have many technical questions about 'no wasting' and you want more details of how to finish the Rectification of the body. Back in Chapter 2 I gave you the 'bendy toy' model of the 'A' frame unblocked structure. So what comes next? What further questions can we have?

SONG

The answer lies in the character 'Song'. We have recognised the vertical axis and discussed the implications. We have looked at the relationship of the limbs to the spine – specifically to the elbows and knees. We have been able to discuss the mechanics of efficient breathing and the need for relaxation. However, we need to clarify just what we mean by relaxation. What exactly are we doing when we relax in Taiji? The classical texts give the answer in the character 'Song'. The Masters give the instruction 'Relax!' and often sigh in frustration at Western students' inability to produce what the Master is looking for.

So, is there any reason to suppose that there could be different understandings of the idea of relaxation? In the West we tend to be very active, striving and struggling, so that when we do something, we try hard. When we think of relaxation, we tend to go to the other extreme. To us, relaxation is going limp, dozing off in the sun, drinking a can of beer, flat out on the sofa, watching the telly.

There appears to be a fairly obvious mismatch between these ideas of relaxation and the type that prevents wasting of Qi. First, if we relax so much that we go limp and collapse in a heap, then we will almost certainly run a risk of blocking Qi. Second, if Qi Gong is supposed to be about moving and living, then this is almost impossible if we are an immobile blob of relaxation. So, if that idea of relaxation is inappropriate, what are the Chinese trying to tell us?

The character 'Song', like all Chinese characters, is a picture, and the idea it depicts is that of loosening, unbinding or slackening off a tie. This means reducing the tension in a binding, not cutting all connections. Most of us have had the experience of sitting for a long time on a journey and having the blood pool in our feet, causing them to swell and making our shoes uncomfortably tight. One response to this is to untie our shoelaces. If we undo them completely and open the front of our shoes, this is the equivalent of relaxing in front of the telly, or lying on the beach relaxed. But what happens when we have to get up and walk? If we leave our shoes undone, they might fall off, so we retie our laces. This time our laces will be less tight. We have 'Song-ed' them. We have loosened, not completely undone or cut them. Alternatively think of the feeling you get when you slip into a hot bath after coming in from a very cold outside. The 'Ahhhh' of feeling yourself releasing into the warmth is feeling 'Song'. Of course most of us stay in the bath way past 'Song' and get really floppy relaxed. But the initial letting go is 'Song'.

'SONG' IS THE EXPRESSION OF TAIJI IN THE BODY

Our Western attitude to relaxation is too near to cutting the laces to help us to find 'Song'. Chinese ideas of relaxation are developed from a consideration of the meaning of Taiji in Yin–Yang philosophy. Taiji is the first state of manifestation realised by the pregnant void, Wuji. In Taiji the emptiness of Wuji is full of Yin and Yang but they are not separated into Yin *and* Yang. In Taiji they are present but totally and harmoniously mixed, balanced and intertwined, presenting only oneness, Taiji.

From this, we can realise that the Taiji in the body cannot be the cut, or limp state, of complete, collapsed relaxation. That would be all Yin, or certainly not have a sufficient balance of Yang to be considered Taiji. On the other hand, it is correct to realise that an excess of tension and activity is too Yang, without a harmonious balance of Yin, to be called a bodily expression of Taiji.

Since activity and its associated tensions are inevitable, we do need to learn to relax, to be less Yang, in order to approach a physical expression of Taiji. However, the limp collapse that is total relaxation means we have overshot our goal of Taiji and simply swapped our Yang for Yin. Bluntly put, we must not relax too much, which brings us back to 'Song' with its implication of not letting go completely.

So we must not relax too much. But how much is too much? As we are all different, the right amount for me may not be the right amount for you or for anyone else. How can we know what is the correct amount? The short answer is that we can know by feeling. More specifically, there is a technique, known as 'testing', that we can use to know the right direction in which to go. Of course, before testing can be of much use we need to have done enough practice to have something to test. A skilful teacher may be able to coax a student into a sufficiently Natural posture that testing this may surprise the student to find how much 'strength' may be found in relaxation. However, initially this is rather more evidence of the teacher's skill than the student's accomplishment. Such experiences engineered by the skilful teacher are provided to motivate students into making the necessary effort at their own personal accomplishment.

TESTING

I am inclined to think that this technique stands almost alone as the most precious of all the treasures hidden in the house of Qi Gong and Taijiquan. For me it has been, and still is, the bridge between practice, the classical writings and philosophy, and my growing experience of Taiji through the practice of Taijiquan.

There is one very important thing to understand about testing. To many people, the word conjures up memories of school and images of passing and failing. The very idea can make us nervous. You might like to think of it as checking if that makes you feel more comfortable. However, we test things all the time to check if they are OK. A photographer looks through the viewfinder to check his composition. The picture that will be produced was, therefore, tested, before using real film, by the look through the viewfinder.

A cook may taste the seasoning of a dish several times before being satisfied with the flavour. Each taste is a test. When arranging flowers, stamps or any collection, we pause from time to time to view the arrangement. Each pause for a look is a test. Testing in Qi Gong practice, be it Taijiquan or any other system, is a pause to view how our practice is developing. This pause for testing, which is like a snapshot of our current development, gives us information to guide our future practice.

This is typical of Chinese pragmatism and empiricism. Do all the verbal explanations really make any difference? The only way to find out is to 'suck it and see'. Bluntly, if knowledge is real, it must make a difference. The only way to find out is to test. How many things do we believe, or think we believe, that we have never tested to see if they really make a difference in our life?

METHODS OF TESTING

In principle anything can be tested, and it is just a question of finding an appropriate method. For visual arrangements, like displays or photographs, the appropriate test is by looking, whilst for flavours it is to taste. If we are building a bridge and we want to test the design, we might make various calculations of loads and stresses against the known strengths of the building materials. Some people seem to think that this method of testing, using measurement and calculation, is in some way superior to other methods. This is misguided.

Measurement and calculation are useful in certain circumstances and irrelevant in others. What possible measurement and calculations could the cook make that would be more efficient than using the magnificent sensitivity of the body? A mechanical series of tests to bring the taste into line with some defined standard is absurd. Why on earth go to all that trouble when our own taste buds can do the job more effectively and efficiently? To insist that the mechanical or mathematical test is more valid is to reveal a poor grasp of reality, and an unhealthy alienation from one's own physical being.

Tension and relaxation are both feelings, so to balance Yin and Yang and express Taiji in the body must also be a feeling. From this, it obviously follows that the appropriate test will be a test that involves feeling, and the Classical Taijiquan verses stress sensitivity, not force.

So what is this feeling and how do we test our practice and current level of achievement? In a book, it is very difficult to tell you and it is also difficult to explain testing in such a way that some people might not make mistakes. Well, here goes anyway.

TESTING 'SONG'

Have you ever slipped slowly into a hot bath on a cold day and enjoyed feeling the heat relaxing you? In the first few moments, we feel the release caused by the heat sinking into our cold body. When we are cold, we tend, unconsciously, to tense up. Sinking into a hot bath, we can feel all our joints relaxing and it feels like our body is expanding. That first release is Song.

The test we use is based on our idea of Rectification. If our Rectification is truly in the direction of harmony with the Laws of Heaven and Earth, then we should find that the Rectified body is stronger and more relaxed – Song – than the unrectified body.

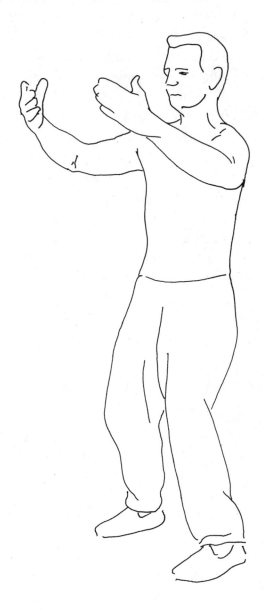

Standing to cultivate 'Song', inner structure and 'No blocking, no wasting'

Simply, the testee stands with the vertical axis extended – head suspended, weight on the tail bone (which incidentally we can now recognise as Song in the spine or back) – and with the four limbs rounded out like a four-legged animal with the knees and elbows being the 'four corners' of the spine/limbs structure.

This rounding out must be 'Song' or 'released' to ensure that there is no blocking in the shoulders or hips. This is definitely not floppy but directed out from the torso in a very specific way. A major way to ensure this outward movement, without trying too hard, is to imagine a flow of Qi to the elbows and knees coming from the flow up and down the spine.

Now, while the testee maintains their felt awareness of this position, the tester puts pressure – at first lightly and later more strongly – to see how the testee feels.

To the person doing this, the testee should feel remarkably firm and stable. The person being tested may be very surprised at how little effect the pressure is having. Frequently, they may ask if their partner is applying any pressure at all, or if they are really trying. This is the first level of testing, static testing, described in Chapter 3. The slowly increasing pressure from the tester acts as a form of amplification for the feelings of the testee. The tester temporarily increases the feedback we all are continuously getting from our bodies' felt sense of being.

The acid test is if the person being tested can smile. Often, people find testing a pleasant experience and smile spontaneously, but a good test is always: Can I smile in this situation of being literally under pressure, being tested? Remember the old doctor in Beijing who laughingly teased me about my too-serious attitude to life by telling me that smiling is also a form of Qi Gong.

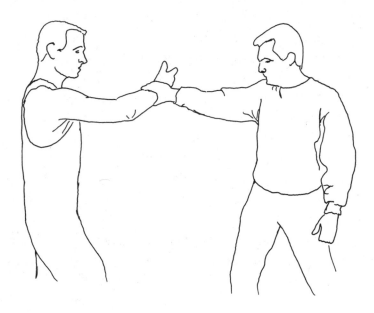

Testing posture to check structure

With a little practice we will find that we can tell very easily if we are coping well or poorly with the test. Through our felt sense of our body, we will know. This method of feeling and testing solves the problem previously raised of knowing when we are relaxed enough but not too much. We do not need to wait twenty or thirty years to know if our practice is doing us any good or worth anything at all. With testing we can feel how we are doing.

Testing is always important, but particularly so in the early days of practice. It is a method of training our feeling and sensitivity. Without testing, the mind can run riot and we can generate for ourselves all sorts of 'feelings' of Qi, which are nothing but delusion. Testing is the method that helps to bring all the words down to earth. Early testing needs to be quite gentle; as we progress we can turn up the volume.

Only testing can help us tell the difference between the accurate sensations of our physical being, which are useful, and self-delusion. There is a danger, however, that testing might become an end in itself, or a source of wasting. The tester must realise that their job is to help the testee, not to make them feel shoved around. The testee must understand that the feelings are more important than not being moved. It cannot be repeated too often that testing is ongoing, with the pressure from the tester acting as a sort of amplifier for the testee's felt sense of the body. It also acts as a reality test to protect us from self-delusion.

Some people, after years of practice with no testing, may be able to convince themselves that they have all sorts of exotic Qi sensations. Such people may be very surprised to discover that all they have got is 'Flower fists and brocade legs'. Pretty to look at perhaps, but empty where the internal feelings are not felt or understood. Our experience of our feelings needs to be trained, just as we train our hands to produce the letter shapes used in writing. Just as we learn to walk, talk and move, we need to learn to feel. That does not mean that we do not feel already, any more than a newborn infant is blind. But, just as the infant must learn to see and recognise particular patterns of light and dark as faces, and as people like mother and father, we need to learn to recognise particular patterns of feeling and their significance.

Testing the vertical axis, the two 'A' frames core of the Rectification of the body, allows us to learn what is the right amount of relaxation for us to operationalise Song in each individual and personal case. It does not matter that this is non-verbal, as long as it is personally recognisable. What can be recognised can be repeated. This allows for development over time and the sensations become more easily repeated on demand.

Once Song has been recognised, we can then go further and extend out to the fingers and toes from the ridgepole and 'A' frame core. After all, we need to include the whole body, not just the spine and limbs down to elbows and knees. Beginners who are still learning Song will have to accept the correct positioning of the forearms and hands, and the lower legs and feet, but this acceptance should never be blind obedience. Anything that your teacher says must be accepted as a working hypothesis, to be tested in experience and practice. You can only progress through your own efforts to internalise and realise what your teacher says.

The body is a unity. Language cuts it to pieces for convenience but in reality you are not an assemblage of separate parts. People are grown. We are continually engaged in 'growing' ourselves out of the ongoing flux of the wave of the moment. This is the wonder of the 'soft' machine. Mechanical devices are assemblages of separate parts, but while 'soft' machines may be fragmented into limbs and organs, they are not assembled from parts to make wholes. Throughout its existence, the living creature – the 'soft' machine – is continuously a whole. To the Chinese, this is the idea of One Qi that permeates, defines and sustains a living creature.

MAKING THE MOST OF YOUR TEACHER

I once attended a seminar by a prominent Taijiquan teacher, who had flown in especially to give this course. We were waiting for the teacher to arrive and the sense of anticipation in the room could almost be felt. He arrived a little late, due to traffic problems. This just raised the tension as the participants waited. At last, the teacher arrived. Now we could begin and everyone in the room directed their attention, eagerly awaiting the first thing that the teacher would say.

'Good morning. I'm sorry I was a little late and I thank you for waiting so patiently. The first thing I want to say is that I can't teach you Taiji.' What? You mean after all this waiting and wanting, you're telling us that you can't teach? What are we all doing here? Should we go now? Should we ask for our money back? What a disappointment! Incidentally, how poor is our Taiji that a few words can switch us so quickly from the Yang of anticipation to the Yin of disappointment. Certainly we were not manifesting Taiji as the point of balance and harmony, the still point in the centre of the cyclone.

Having paused for long enough for us to have our reactions to the first words, the teacher continued, 'I can't teach you Taiji because I can't teach you anything. You can *learn* Taiji. I can show you my realisation of Taiji. I can talk to you about Taiji. I can even suggest various postures, exercises and tricks that I have found useful in my study. They may or may not be useful or effective for you. I can only talk, show and share with you. You all learn from your own experience. Your experience is your teacher, not me.'

The best a teacher can do is show you. Sometimes, this can involve adjusting your position, correcting you a bit, or a lot. You must then take what your teacher gives you and run with it. Only when you make the understanding your own, can you, and you alone, do the fine-tuning that is necessary. As I am fond of saying to my own students, 'It's your body not mine. I might be able to move you along a bit but only you can know for sure.'

The teacher also has another function. Teachers are our inspiration. They show us that the study is worthwhile and produces definite benefits. They can do things that we cannot. All practitioners who succeed in their study and practice can be inspirations and living yardsticks.

However, just because someone has great accomplishment, this does not mean that they can automatically teach. Teaching is like gardening, as indeed is study. The Chinese specifically refer to Qi Gong in general as a 'way of self cultivation'. Just because someone is a good gardener in their own allotment does not necessarily mean that they can help someone else cultivate another allotment with different soil. A teacher must minimally have sufficient accomplishment to be capable of being a living inspiration, as well as sufficient experience of study to be familiar with the learning process.

However, even with an excellent teacher, progress will only come from your own efforts. As Liang Tsung Tsai wrote:

If you rely too much on teachers – best have no teacher.

If you rely too much on books – best read no book.

(Liang 1977)

SUMMARY

So what is the final position for Rectification of the body? How are the legs and arms arranged? The answer lies in three parts:

First   No blocking or wasting

Second   The ridge pole – 'A' frame basic pattern

Third   Song in all directions

We must remember that we are three-dimensional beings, so we have to release or 'Song' all our joints in all directions. This is the meaning of being round, a common injunction in Qi Gong systems and also in Taijiquan.

The Rectified body is both the requirement for, and the product of, a unified One Qi, that is circulating freely, not blocked or wasted anywhere. There are two ways to describe the basic standing posture of this Rectified body. One uses the observable relationships between specific points on the body surface. The other uses mental images as descriptions of sensations. The difference between these two is that the first is quantitative, while the second is qualitative.

An appropriately labelled illustration of a posture will show the observable structural relationships but may be of very little use in helping people control it. With some experience of relating what a posture feels like to what it looks like, most people then find pictures are informative but not necessarily instructive.

Advice using images can be confusing if the context is not clear. When we use an image to convey what something is *like*, we need to know what it is about the image that matters. Suppose that we were looking at several cars of different colours. If I said that one reminded me of a banana, I doubt you would think I meant in shape. In that context the yellow colour of the banana is what matters. Images used in Taijiquan and Qi Gong teaching must be understood in this context. When the teaching speaks of being 'round like a balloon', it cannot be taken literally. Because we try to Song in all directions, we feel 'round' especially in the sense that we feel *all* of our body from the top of the head, through the back, to the tips of the fingers and toes.

The imagery used expresses both the quality of a posture as it is felt or experienced and also the visual quality of the posture. Whilst the technical details of alignment and co-ordination are important, the qualities, or felt sense, of the posture are of equal importance. Also the harmony of paired opposites must be expressed to qualify as not blocked or wasted – as an expression of Taiji.

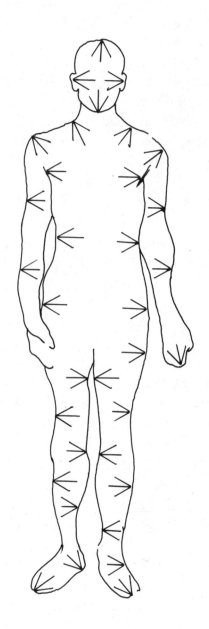

'Song' in all directions: Feeling 'round'

BASIC STANDING POSTURE

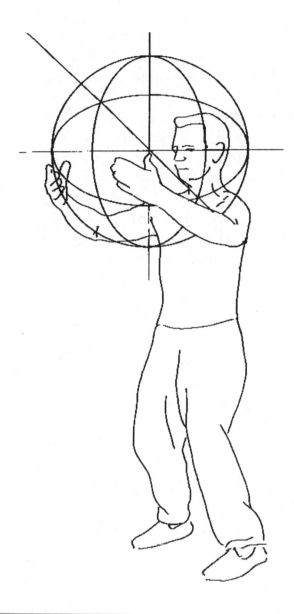

Zhan Zhuang Qi Gong: 'Holding a ball'

The diagram on the previous page shows the basic standing posture common to many forms, schools and styles of Qi Gong. In the Taijiquan of the Yang family, as transmitted by Yang Cheng Fu, via his son Yang Sau-cheng, and his student Chu King Hung, this posture is called Qi Gong. This is not so much a name for the posture but for the activity that is manifested by this posture.

The basic vertical axis is present, which is being gently uplifted from the top – *a light and sensitive energy is placed on the head top* – and gently pulled down at the bottom – *a weight hangs from the tip of the tail bone.* Technically the Ni Wan, or Bai Hui, point on the crown of the skull is positioned such that a tangent to the curve of the skull at that point is parallel to the ground, and the tangent at the Wei Lu point, at the tip of the coccyx, is also parallel to the ground.

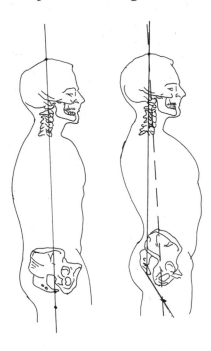

Wei Lu–Ni Wan alignment. Right correct: Ni-wan at the top of the skull is vertically aligned with Wei Lu at the tip of the coccyx; Left incorrect

The knees and elbows are projected in a relaxed fashion 'to the four corners', in keeping with the basic four-limbed pattern we share with all four-legged animals. This produces, with the vertical axis, what we have called the 'ridgepole or "A" frame' alignment.

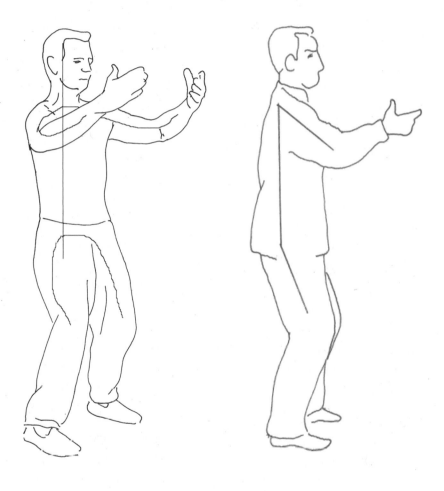

Standing 'A' frame alignment: View 1   *Standing 'A' frame alignment· View 2*

The forearms from the point of the elbow to the middle knuckle, through the wrists, are projected in a continuous line to keep the wrists 'straight'. The fingers are extended, to direct the Qi to the tips of the fingers, and gently spread. This ensures that the hands are Song, too.

The knees are positioned over the toes.

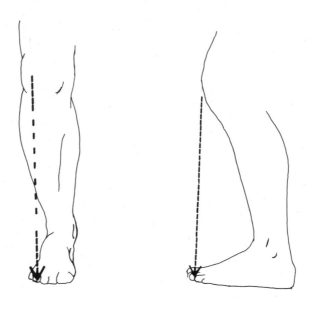

Knee over toe: third or 'ring' toe is correct. Front view — Yang on outside, Yin on inside; side view — Yang surface

Specifically, the point of the knee is held vertically above the 'ring' toe, i.e. counting the big toe as one, the fourth toe next to the little toe. The feet are flat and relaxed with the weight in the ball, heel and outside edge of the foot. Technically, the Yong Quan point in the sole of the foot is the root or focus of the weight but the distribution must be even in the areas described. The weight of the body runs down the outside, or Yang surface, of the leg.

THREE CIRCLE THEORY

The legs and arms must be round because of Song in three dimensions. The way to cultivate this roundness is to feel round. Specifically, we should feel a ball between the legs and in the space embraced by the arms. The easiest way to get this round, ball-like feeling is to use what is called 'Three Circle Theory'.

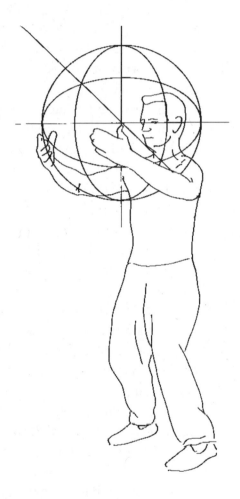

Zhan Zhuang Qi Gong: 'Holding a ball'

We work to visualise and feel the three circles at right angles that describe the balls embraced by the arms and between the knees. These three circles can be called flat circle, side circle and front circle. When standing in this posture, we work to feel all three circles for each ball and to make them all the same diameter. Testing at intervals can be very helpful here to help check any biases to favouring a particular circle.

Standing in this posture, or more realistically, learning how to stand in this posture and feel it intimately, is both a form of meditation and Qi Gong. The meditative aspect comes from the necessary mental state to feel and image the posture fully. The mind becomes absorbed in the posture and settles into the body. This is a sign that Taiji is being approached. The Yin–Yang of mind and body melt into undifferentiated unity. Both are present, but so intimately associated and so well harmonised that neither Yin nor Yang, body or mind, are discernible, only the unity of Taiji. Just standing like this is both the practice and the realisation of Taiji and Qi Gong. As the body relaxes and the separation between mind and body dissolves, the natural wave of movement due to breathing spreads out through the entire body. The whole body breathes. This is movement in stillness.

However, this is difficult and, for many beginners, virtually impossible to achieve or maintain for any period of time. For this reason, many varieties of patterns of movement have been developed to make it easier for the mind to stay involved with the body. In Taijiquan, in particular, we find the famous slow motion 'shadow boxing' forms or routines. These are often called stillness in movement. What is it that is still? They are also called moving Qi Gong. How is that?

The answers to both questions come from the maintenance of the Rectified body alignment and relationships throughout the movement. It is the basic pattern or structure that is 'still'. The adoption and realisation of this body condition, in movement with mental attention, is Qi Gong, hence moving Qi Gong.

Chapter 6 | Methods and Techniques

The last two chapters have been about what I call the 'Rectification' of the body. In Qi Gong circles, it is usually expressed as working to ensure 'No blocking, no wasting' of Qi. A more general Chinese Natural Science view, favoured by doctors, biologists and those seeking for longevity, or immortality, would be 'returning to nature'. In the Yang family transmission, it is also called 'Three Circle Theory'.

None of these groups would be particularly uncomfortable with calling it the physical expression of Taiji, which is not the same as the art of Taijiquan. This might be confusing for those of you who habitually use the Western abbreviation of Taijiquan, and call your practice Tai Chi. Chinese are very frequently confused by Westerners who use this contraction.

TAIJI AND TAIJIQUAN ARE NOT THE SAME

There are many different 'Quan', literally a 'fist'. When it is used in the name of an art, or system of techniques, I suppose the handiest translation is 'boxing'. This is not quite all the story. First, virtually all 'Quan' employ various techniques, not just boxing and the use of fists. Second, 'Quan' are the national sport or pastimes of China, and the overtones of meaning include ideas similar to our ideas about sport. So, 'Quan' can mean 'fist', 'boxing' and 'physical excellence, or discipline'.

Taiji, however, is a more philosophical idea. It is represented by the Taiji Tu, or Yin/Yang diagram. This is becoming increasingly familiar outside China and is a circle divided by a reverse 'S' into two halves. Usually, one is white and the other black and each half contains a dot of the other's colour. The two shapes look a little like two fishes swimming in a circle, chasing each other. It represents a perfectly harmonious blending of Yin and Yang into unity, Taiji.

Translating the characters 'Taiji' is tricky. 'Ji' originally meant 'the ridgepole of a tent'. Later its meaning was extended to 'crossroads', 'junction' or 'place where things meet or come together' and so it is even used to describe a railway junction or terminus. 'Tai' on its own is fairly easy. It means 'biggest' or 'greatest'. We have even borrowed it into English in our word 'typhoon', which in Chinese is 'Tai Feng' or 'greatest wind'. When 'Tai' and 'Ji' are combined in 'Taiji', the literal translations are all clumsy, 'grand terminus', 'supreme ultimate' and so on. These might appeal to the romantics among us but they are not exactly clear.

My personal favourite is to compare 'Taiji' to our own idea of the 'still point in the centre of the cyclone'. Some people may like to use the word 'God' as a translation for 'Taiji' in its universal aspect. As long as you do not think of God as some type of 'gaseous celestial invertebrate', I will not argue with you. But it should be remembered that we can also have non-universal aspects of Taiji. Just as we can talk about Yin and Yang as universal principles, we can also have *particular* Yin–Yang relationships such as body–mind, dark–light and the much overused female–male.

A healthy nation would be one which is a Taiji of the Yin of the people and the Yang of the state. A healthy landscape achieves Taiji of the Yin of the earth with the Yang of civilisation. This seems a particularly appropriate Taiji for us to aim at when confronting problems like global warming. Thus, a healthy body is one in which Yin and Yang are unified into Taiji. The body, Yin, and the mind, Yang, are harmonised. The feeling, Xin, is Yin relative to the intention, Yi, which is Yang, which gives us another human Taiji.

Taijiquan is a physical discipline of 'boxing', that is a vehicle for approaching Taiji through the achievement of various smaller human Taiji-s. It is a way of expressing and experiencing the idea, Taiji. When you move through the postures of a Taijiquan round, you simultaneously demonstrate your current grasp of Taiji and have the opportunity to expand that knowledge.

So, achieving 'No blocking, no wasting' of your Qi, while it is *a* Taiji, is only a beginning method of Taijiquan, a foundation method. I have discussed it mostly in static postures because that is the easiest way to describe it. It cannot, for Taijiquan players, really be separated from the movements of that art. But this initial method of Rectification needs to be understood before the famous slow motion shadow boxing can be well practised.

DAOYIN

After the method of Rectification comes the method of Daoyin. In your practice it can be very difficult to separate these two as each of them feeds the other. Daoyin can be used to achieve Rectification, but Rectification is a prerequisite of Daoyin. The two really go hand in hand for Taijiquan players. It is only for ease of communication that the two are split.

WHAT ARE METHODS AND TECHNIQUES?

I distinguish between methods and techniques to try and clarify some confusions that arise. A method is a set of principles that we are trying to realise and express. A technique is the vehicle that we use for realisation and expression.

It is not uncommon for the Chinese to say confusing things like:

> All martial and therapeutic arts and exercises are Qi Gong.

> Taijiquan and Xingyiquan are internal while The Eight Pieces of Brocade and Shaolin Temple Boxing are external. But they are both the same.

> In the Internal, from soft to hard; in the External, from hard to soft.

What on earth can they mean? How can they say that they are the same? What does internal – soft to hard – and external – hard to soft – mean?

What the Chinese are saying is that the method is, at bottom, the same but that the techniques used along the way by different schools and styles may differ. That the goal is the same is reflected by the internal/external conclusion of both resulting in hard and soft together. That the techniques differ is encapsulated by the tag, 'internal – soft to hard; external – hard to soft'.

We can use cooking as an analogy to assist our understanding. Cooking is a method of preparing food to eat and so sustain life. Different national and regional styles of cooking are techniques to produce specific types of dishes. As long as the balance of essential ingredients for nourishment are present, we can live just as easily on a diet prepared according to English, French, Chinese or Indian techniques. Given exactly the same ingredients, different meals will be produced by different cooks, using different techniques. Since the ingredients are the same, the nourishment will be comparable. The taste and texture may be very different but the food value will be the same. Similarly, the Chinese tend to discuss their exercise systems in terms of the 'taste' or 'flavour' of each.

PEOPLE ARE INDIVIDUALS, UNIQUE AND DIFFERENT

Just as particular foods or dishes are more appropriate at different times of day or for different types of people, so different techniques are more, or less, suited to different people. Patients recovering from a heart attack need exercise to recover effectively. However, few people would suggest that such patients should enter a marathon or climb a mountain straight away.

We are all aware that other people differ from us. We have different coloured hair, eyes, skin colour and different heights, weights and body types. Given such wide variety on the outside, it is incredible that we should think that we are identical on the inside and that we all need identical diets or exercise plans.

Such thinking is too crude and specific. We can say that we all need to harmonise with the Laws of Heaven and Earth and we need to not block or waste Qi. However, these statements, while general enough to be true for everyone, do not generate specific end states that are identical for everyone. One person's meat can be another's poison, as the English proverb goes. Each of us has a unique inner nature and its expression is the achievement of harmony.

DAOYIN IS QI GONG

Qi Gong is 'effort, work or exercise on that which is essential to life'. Everything that is life enhancing can legitimately be called Qi Gong. All medicine, diet, exercises and breathing are Qi Gong. One could almost translate Qi Gong as general health preservation and maintenance. This is why the Chinese can happily call all therapeutic exercise Qi Gong, and then go even further and say that acupuncture is Qi Gong, medicine is Qi Gong, diet is Qi Gong and, even, 'smiling is a form of Qi Gong'.

However, such a general term can easily be confusing. Different terms have been used at different times in Chinese history to specifically refer to exercises that are Qi Gong. Overall the three most common have been Qi Gong, Tu Na and Daoyin.

Tu Na, which literally means inhalation–exhalation, was popular at one time. This captures the control of the breathing that is an important aspect of Chinese therapeutic exercise. However, this over-emphasises breathing at the expense of the rest of the body and can lead to all sorts of troubles.

Daoyin is the term for these Qi Gong exercises that I personally prefer, since it captures the principles we are trying to realise most succinctly. Daoyin has been translated as 'the way of nurture', 'the way of Yin', and 'guiding and inducing'. It consists of two characters, Dao (Tao), the Way, and Yin, the opposite of Yang. The easiest way to grasp the meaning of Daoyin is by an analogy and the traditional image is of melt water from a snow-capped mountain running down in the spring.

First of all, the water does not run any old way. The Chinese reject the idea of randomness in the universe. Water always flows downhill along the path of least resistance. It finds its Way, its Tao (Dao). This Way then guides the water.

However, it is the nature of water to both dissolve (it is called the universal solvent) and to erode. These characteristics of water mean that, over time, its Way becomes enhanced. The tiny trickle flowing along a slight irregularity in the mountain surface grows and becomes a stream, then it becomes a river, possibly ending up as large as the Grand Canyon.

This is Daoyin, the guiding of the flow of water. The flowing induces, or nurtures, the guide way and thus becomes stronger. This is the Way of Yin or the way of nurture. Yin follows, and hence is passive, but it produces something, for Yin is also nurturing or fertile. Yin is the womb that produces the next generation by receiving the active trigger of the Yang sperm, but the passivity of Yin is illusory. Yin nurtures and develops the Yang spark to allow the new birth to be made manifest in the world.

DAOYIN AND GONG FU: INTERNAL AND EXTERNAL

But what is guided and induced? Since Daoyin, Qi Gong and Tu Na are all synonyms, the guiding and inducing must have something to do with both Qi and inhalation–exhalation. It is at this point that the internal and external schools temporarily part company.

The externalists tend to practise techniques of movement and breathing, just as the teacher shows it. The guide comes from the teacher, hence is external, and the inducing is often very strenuous. In external styles the teacher bears a great responsibility to ensure that students are following the correct techniques to guide their Qi and breathing and that the rate of induction is not so fast as to lead to problems.

After long practice, the students will begin to feel the Qi flow in their bodies, which is the real source of the techniques.

They can then move on from the mechanical techniques of movement to the internal sensations of the flow of movement, hence from hard to soft. This approach suits younger, or more impatient, students who want to 'get stuck in' and feel that they are 'getting somewhere'. It can be described as being body conditioning first, generating internal awareness of Qi second.

The internalists are encouraged to try and sense the natural tendencies to movement inherent in the body and then use these as guides to movement. This explains the emphasis placed on sensitivity in Taijiquan and other internal systems. Here, of course, the techniques emerge from the nurturing of the natural tendencies to move, the flow of Qi. From an awareness of Qi develops the conditioning of the body, hence from soft to hard. This approach suits those students who are older or convalescent, and thus less initially robust. Because of this, they have more patience and sensitivity. Such students are less concerned about getting somewhere, or getting 'stuck in'. They are more willing to simply be interested in what they are doing right now.

In practice, the differences are not as great as might at first appear. Few internal students start their studies with the sensitivity required to find these natural tendencies to movement, which can then allow them to guide their bodies' movements and so nurture or induce greater flow of Qi. Most internal students have to take their guides from the teacher, just as the external stylists do. The difference is that the internal teacher will try to help students realise that the movements are expressions of Qi flow and the internal student will pay close attention to the movements, trying to find the natural flow of Qi that is hidden in the technique or movement.

The internal school is Yin, relatively speaking, since the internal way is to nurture Qi and encourage it to grow at a rate that is harmonious with the individual students' current level of achievement. The external school is Yang, relatively speaking, since it stimulates development through impositions from outside and is less sensitive to the individual student. Here it is the teacher, rather than the student, who bears the responsibility for the safe assessment of the suitable rate of development and increased intensity of practice.

Both schools have their place and value but both have their own areas of weakness, which can lead to degenerative practices. The internal can become sloppy or lazy, an excuse for not challenging yourself sufficiently for growth to occur. It can also lead to sloth, as well as spiritual, mental and emotional delusions. The external can become simply brutal and strenuous, resulting in emotional insensitivity as well as physical and mental harm. Additionally, in both systems the student is always dependent on the teacher and can rarely progress faster than the teacher is willing to allow. The teacher remains the gatekeeper of the knowledge contained in the particular system and approach.

At present in the West, while external schools frequently struggle with a bad press, the internal schools seem to be more degenerate in their understanding and practice. There are excellent internal teachers but they are far less common than their external counterparts. Even allowing for the occasional rogue external teacher or student, the external schools are of generally higher quality than the internal. This is a great pity, since the internal, with its emphasis on self-paced learning and study, is potentially more widely applicable than the external, which requires either established robustness or youth to develop it.

The problem for the internalists is neatly encapsulated in the Taijiquan proverb 'First in the mind and then in the body'. Understanding is an essential prerequisite to internal study. There is an anonymous verse in the Yang family collection of Taijiquan writings that says, 'To learn something good you have to use your mind a little.' This understanding is not that easy to communicate in its native tongue, so consider how much more difficult it must be for a non-Chinese speaker.

DAOYIN IN TAIJIQUAN

This brings me back to Daoyin – guiding and inducing. First, we must find the guide and then we must follow it. Deliberately tracing out the guides, both mentally and physically, helps to 'dredge the channels', thereby increasing Qi circulation by improving the signal to noise ratio and channel capacity.

However, and this cannot be over-emphasised, the body should be as near as possible to a Rectified condition so that the Natural guides can be clearly sensed and followed. There is a not infrequent tradition that internal styles are learnt after the external has been pursued for some time. I suspect that the necessity for an unblocked and non-wasted body is part of the reason behind this tradition. External training is not necessarily a prerequisite but the awareness of body principles, Rectification, is necessary.

In practice there is a very strong relationship and overlap between Rectification and Daoyin. The guiding and inducing will help to correct posture as the Qi is developed and unified. However, if body principles of Rectification are not adhered to, it is possible to lock the Qi into poor circulation, which may actually cause ill health. Simply, if you are not clear inside, or as clear as you can be, then you will not be able to feel the guides and hence unable to follow them.

AN EXERCISE TO LEARN DAOYIN

To teach the practice of Daoyin, I use the following exercise. In a sense, almost any pattern of movement that is designed according to the principle of 'No blocking, no wasting' can be used. The simpler the exercise, the better for beginners, so I use a simple arm-flapping breathing exercise.

Stand with your feet about shoulder width apart. Minimally the feet must be straight ahead, parallel and at least the width of the pelvis apart. Start at the top of your head. Suspend your head from the ceiling – place a light and sensitive energy at the head top, pigtail tied to the rafters, head floating on the neck. Very often, what we think is vertical is not. To make sure that your head is on straight, you need to locate the point Yu Chen (Jade Pillow).

This is easy. Push your chin forward and block your neck. Feel at the base of your skull at the back. You will find the bulge of the back of your skull and underneath it a dent or hollow, caused by pushing your chin forward. Put a finger gently into this hollow. As you push the top of your head gently upwards, bring your chin back in towards your throat.

You will be able to feel your skull rotating forwards. Keep your finger pressed up towards the skull but let the skull rotate. You will feel the hollow filling out. It feels like the skin is being stretched over the hollow like a drum or tambourine. Just at the base of the skull, when the chin has swung in enough for the skin over the hollow to feel firm but not tight, taut or tense, you will feel a dip or cavity called 'xue' by the acupuncturists. This particular one is Yu Chen – the Jade Pillow – because it is where you place a Chinese jade pillow if you are using one.

To be confident that your head is on straight, feel the 'up' lift from the top of the head (Bai Hui) and then hang your body underneath your head. To help the neck to hang straight, feel the Jade Pillow full and pressed gently back and up. Never try too hard, tense the neck or in any way stiffen it. *Feel* the lift and the full Yu Chen, don't try to do it. Imagine it if you cannot feel it.

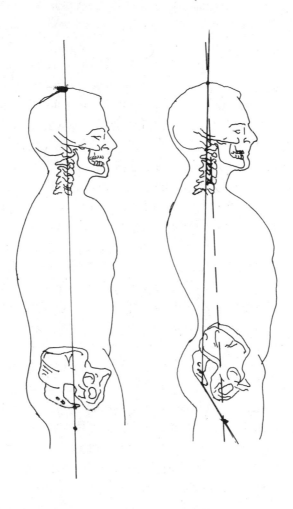

Yu Chen at the base of the skull and Wei Lu point located on the tip of the coccyx

With the head up and the neck straight, the whole body can 'hang' from the head like a puppet. To help this, feel a weight attached to the very tip of your coccyx (tail bone). This weight, in combination with the suspended head top, gently stretches and lengthens the spine, allowing the pelvis to swing freely down and forwards. The pelvis becomes perfectly horizontal and can now act as a bowl to support the contents of the torso.

While it is possible to achieve this spinal extension with straight legs, most people find it easier to allow the vertical pull down on the tail to push the knees forwards, as the pelvis swings into its place. The knees move forwards and slightly outward to come over the 'ring' toe. The groin and hips relax – 'Song' – to allow the legs to become 'round' and balanced, according to the Three Circle Theory.

All of this should be familiar as Rectifying the body, especially the spine and legs. You must not force this posture. You need to clearly visualise this shape in your mind. Then, using this image, try to get your body to feel like your image. You can use visual clues, especially at first, to look and see if you are straight, or if your knees are moving in the direction needed so that they can arrive over the 'ring' toes.

Sometimes, external information can be very useful. For example, many people tend to lean backwards when they think they feel absolutely vertical. External clues from mirrors, teachers and fellow students can help us to train our feelings to be more accurate. However, it is very important to realise that the usefulness of such external information lies in its ability to help us find the internal feelings and only that. Never use mirrors to force yourself into postures. Check out your feelings from time to time but always create and alter your postures through your feelings and images. Remember it is 'First in the mind and then in the body'.

Now that the vertical axis is corrected, we can move to the arms. Relax, Song your shoulders and place your hands, fingertips touching, at your lower Dantien. Feel as if you have a large ball in your arms and that you are embracing this ball.

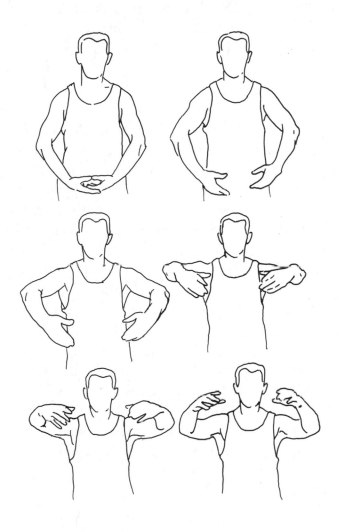

Learning Daoyin Part 1: Arms floating

Relax your shoulder blades against your back by feeling a space under your armpits. Let your elbows spring gently forwards. Keep your shoulders down, and slightly forwards. All this is to get 'Three Circles' in your arms, with your hands at your lower Dantien.

So far, all that I have written is to get your body into an open, unblocked and not wasted condition. Take a moment to relax and sink into this posture. Sink your Qi into your lower Dantien, and fix your breathing at this point. Become as Song as you are able. Relax, unbind and try as little as possible – 'Wei Wu-Wei'. Hang loose and open – round.

Make your breathing long, slow, smooth, fine and deep. Listen to your breathing. Let it become silent, or at least quiet. Stay aware of your breathing and pay attention to your elbows. If you are open, unblocked and Song, not wasted, you will be able to feel a slight tendency to move in your elbows. As you breathe in, they lift and open more forwards; as you breathe out they sink back to their starting point. Different people may describe this feeling in a variety of ways. Perhaps it feels like bellows under your armpits and upper arms or maybe like wings gently flapping. It does not matter what words or images you use, as long as they make sense to you and you can use them to tune into your felt sense of your body and its movement.

Keep paying attention to this movement. If it is not very strong, you can *gently* flap your elbows. This paying attention, feeling part, is the first half of Daoyin. You are using your Xin, feeling mind, to find the Way of your arms at the elbow. Now visualise the path of the elbows in the air. See it as a line if that helps. Project the little movement forwards along its Natural curve. This is using your Yi, imagination, intention, will.

Finally, guide your elbows along this path. Do not use force. Allow your arms to float gently along their Natural track. Keep feeling them as they move. Pay particular attention to your shoulders, keeping them down and relaxed. As soon as you feel tension in your shoulders, or they start to lift, let your elbows sink back and your curved arms return to their starting point.

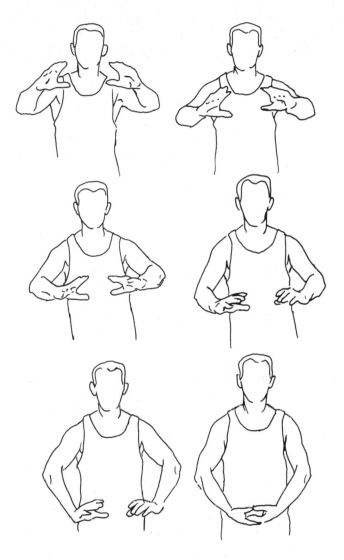

Learning Daoyin Part 2: Arms sinking

Keep repeating this exercise, using your feelings to learn more and more about the tracks of your arms. Use these feelings to make your intention clearer and clearer. Eventually, your arms will move by will alone. They will feel relaxed and heavy.

THE THREE SYSTEMS OF DAOYIN QI GONG

Three systems are important in Daoyin Qi Gong (guiding–inducing Qi work):

- the mind

- the body

- the breathing.

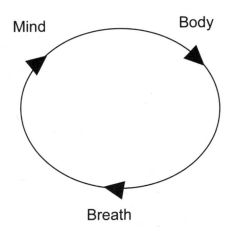

The three systems required for Daoyin/Qigong

These are cyclically inter-related; the mind guides the body through particular patterns of movement. The mind *induces* movement. The movement guides respiration to become long, slow, calm and quiet. The body *induces* breathing. The breathing guides the mind into relaxation. The more relaxed and focused the mind becomes, the better it can attend to the body movements. The mental image of the task becomes both more accurate and more detailed. The breathing *induces* mind. The mind can now refine and improve the movement and the cycle repeats.

CONCLUSION

We have now completed the description of the second developmental task of Taijiquan. It is not the second in a linear sense because Taijiquan is a holistic art. It is not even very easy to divide Rectification from Daoyin in practice. The more successful you are at Rectification, the easier you will find Daoyin. It is much easier to find and follow the Qi flows, when blocking and wasting are reduced as much as possible. On the other hand, the more successful you are at Daoyin, the more you will induce a Rectified body.

In traditional schools, younger, or more robust, students are encouraged to use standing postures at the outset of their training to develop their Three Circle (Rectified) body. Traditionally postures may be held for as long as an hour or more. This may seem harsh, but it is because they can more easily adapt to the rigours of such a training technique. Maintaining a posture for Rectification purposes for an extended period of time may be difficult and indeed hard work for many. We are tempted to 'hold' the posture fixed. This is an error and contributes to the problem. It is vital to become 'Fang Song', relax into the posture and allow the structure

147

to maintain itself and gently move with the breath – Jing Gong. I would encourage any serious student to engage with standing practice and stance holding. Build up slowly from 1 minute and then 3 minutes, and then 5 until 15–20 minutes becomes comfortable. The traditional emphasis on extended standing reflects the primacy of this method.

Other students, who lack the robustness of either mind or body to withstand this, can start with moving. However, their practice must be focused on using the Daoyin of moving to reduce blockages and wasting of Qi. Movement must be done 'mindfully', that is with attention. The Xin must feel for the tendencies to move to provide the Yi with the movement template. While the Yi is executing movement the Xin must monitor the movement continuously to further refine the movement template for the next repetition of that move.

We are now beginning to perceive that there is a syllabus of Taijiquan. Whether standing or moving, the first developmental task is Rectification of the body. This can be called the unification of the Qi, returning to nature, or achieving Taiji of mind and body.

If you are teaching beginners, your first obligation is to teach this. The techniques you use may vary according to the students and their capacities. For some, strict standing practice will be appropriate, prior to form practice. For others, gentle movements with much emphasis on 'Song' and 'roundness' – Three Circle Theory – will be more acceptable.

To a certain extent, how long someone stays a 'beginner' depends on how much Rectification is needed and how long this takes. Teachers do not do their students any favours by jumping to 'going with the flow' too soon. Daoyin is indeed the method of 'going with the flow', but, and I cannot emphasise this too strongly, without good teaching and awareness of 'No blocking, no wasting' a serious risk exists that whatever flow is encouraged may be detrimental. This is the risk of locking bad habits, bad posture and bad Qi into yourself and your students.

Only *after* 'Song', 'roundness' and 'No blocking, no wasting' have become automatic can the emphasis shift to Daoyin. Even when Daoyin – guiding and inducing – becomes the focus of practice, we can never afford to neglect or forget Rectification and Three Circle Theory.

Part III

The Art of Taijiquan

Chapter 7 | The Six Secrets

THE SIX SECRETS

In this chapter we will begin to examine what many people see as the art of Taijiquan. I will describe the details of technique, training and performance called the Six Secrets, as handed down in the transmission of Chu King Hung, disciple of Yang Sau-cheng, son of Yang Cheng Fu. Traditionally, the levels of detail and refinement that I am going to cover are not given to students in advance of their personal development. This is in order to not distract students, and to avoid the negative results that might come from attempting something too soon.

In the past the teacher would give the student an instruction and then wait and watch to see if the student worked until flashes of the next level of refinement emerged spontaneously. On seeing these, the teacher would then point them out to the student and give the relevant teaching to further assist the development and expression of this more refined execution of the moves. Then, again, the teacher would settle back to wait and watch for the spontaneous stirrings of the next refinement. This cycle of teacher teaching and student working, learning and developing was the traditional technique. After completing training a student could look back and see the stages of development that had been achieved;

even stages that at the beginning were beyond the level of a beginner's ability to see and understand.

I agree with this traditional position. It is far better to concentrate your practice on your current position than to dream about what you are 'going' to be able to do. If you do not build up from sound basics at a sensible pace, you are never going to be able to do anything fancy. It is also true that violating a developmental chain can result in negative results. It is possible to do Taijiquan in such a misconceived way that you can actually damage the health of your 'bodymind'.

However, while I agree with the traditional reasons, I also see that they do not solve the problems of poor student concentration, or the negative results of poor practice. The traditional silence has resulted in confusion and its attendant problems. Taijiquan players have become separatist and many are over-ready to condemn others whose practice is different. The confusion that currently exists contributes to students being unable to focus their practice effectively.

In Chapter 2 I told the story of the blind men and the elephant and I do not need to go into it again. This book is intended to be my sketch of as much of the 'Taijiquan elephant' as I can see. I do not claim to be able to give you a perfect 3D hologram of it, just my little sketch. The purpose of this book is to allow people to relax, knowing that there is a syllabus. Then, they can get on with their present practice, confident that there will be more to get on with when their bodies are ready.

I accept that there is a risk of encouraging people to get out of their depth. Many people are in a rush. We all tend to belittle what seems simple and pursue what seems advanced but, with the current confusion, sometimes it can be difficult to distinguish between the two. By giving my sketch of the transmission of one Taijiquan school, I hope to reduce such mistakes rather than encourage more.

In the end, my reasons for writing this book are the same as the traditional reasons for silence. The well being of all students everywhere is still the goal. As times change, so do strategies, and what was once appropriate may no longer be so. The lesson of change is the most important lesson to be found in this art. Taijiquan players should be the last people to make the mistake of trying last year's strategy today. Not for us should be the position of the Allied generals at the start of World War II, all ready for trench warfare and completely unprepared for Blitzkrieg. Finally, as Westerners we seem to have more of a need to have things clearly mapped out.

The sequence of training provided by Master Chu King Hung is called the Six Secrets and they are as follows:

1. Three Circle Form

2. Yin–Yang Form

3. Spiral, or Qi, Form

4. Centre-Turn Form

5. Spiral Leg Form

6. Yin–Yang – Head–Hands.

NEI GONG

Nei Gong means 'inner work' in Chinese, and literally refers to breathing exercises for the internal muscles of the body, diaphragm and intercostals. I use this term in a slightly wider sense for I also include the deeper levels of form, the so-called Six Secrets. This is because I emphasise the Rectification of the body as a prerequisite of practice.

I was also taught advanced breathing techniques. These allow you to withstand blows or strikes to the abdomen by encouraging you to 'spread' or 'inflate' your Qi throughout your body. They involve so-called reverse breathing and are a foundation for the development of 'rebound' energy. They also provide the thread, or chain, to bind together the Six Secrets so that finally all that is left is the breathing. These were also taught under the title 'Nei Gong'.

THE SIX SECRETS AS NEI GONG

Until the body is fairly close to its true, or Natural, structure, some of the subtler details of the postures are imperceptible. This is why they are called secrets. Each relies, to some extent, on the development of the others. Until you have learnt to walk, you cannot begin to appreciate running, jumping and dancing. It is the same in the development of your Qi Gong. This parallel between development in the art and in the development from child to adult is one of the reasons Qi Gong and Taijiquan are called ways of self cultivation.

The Rectification of the body is a necessary precursor. It is the framework for the expression and experience of the subtleties of the art, and is expressed in a very particular structure and posture. To develop well, attention must be focused on the bones, joints and muscles. To me, this is clearly external work, so I feel justified in calling the development and detail of internally generated postures, internal work, Nei Gong.

After, and only after, Rectification can Daoyin be a truly reliable way of practice. In the meantime, we have to use a great deal of 'Yi', imagination, intention or will. This is clearly mental effort, and is what is primarily required to develop and evoke the posture from an increasingly Rectified body. It is a job of realising and finding the forms within your own body. It is an *expression* of form, *not* an *imposition*. This mental aspect is also part of my use of Nei Gong.

DISCUSSION OF THE SIX SECRETS

Before we start, I just want to point out that using the word 'secret' does not mean that we are going to go all esoteric and deposit our brains at the door. Anything that you do not know, or is hidden from you, is secret. There are always huge areas of knowledge that are only known by a few people. So much of life is a secret. Electronic engineering, or even the wiring in your home, can be a secret. How my car works is mostly secret from me.

I believe that all of these secrets are available for me to understand, if I take the time. The information is not hidden, but unless I take the trouble to learn, it will remain secret. Even with study, many areas have 'trade' secrets that are not necessarily in the books because you cannot appreciate their worth or necessity until after you have learnt the basics.

The Taijiquan secrets are a mix of both. In the past they have been hidden by virtue of not being widely publicised. They are also secrets because of their developmental character. Until we evolved to stand on two legs, we needed our arms to support us. So, much manual activity would have remained secret.

1. THREE CIRCLE THEORY

Three Circle Theory is essentially the same as what I call Rectification of the body. It is the expression and cultivation of 'No blocking, no wasting'. By expressing three circles in the arms and legs, while at the same time hanging from the head with a weight on the tail bone, 'No blocking, no wasting' and Rectification are achieved. Master Chu characterised the initial learning of the long form, from Yang Sau-cheng, as learning 'Three Circle Form'. His emphasis was to perform the form 'Fang Song' or relaxed and rounded with the correct alignment of knees, elbows, hips, shoulders, hands and feet. The previous chapters have covered this foundational aspect in great detail so we do not need to go into it all again here.

2. YIN–YANG FORM

All of Qi Gong, traditional Chinese medicine (TCM) and high culture are thoroughly filled with Yin–Yang theory. So, in one sense, it seems odd to find it as a particular topic. The Chinese will very happily smile, nod and say, 'Well, of course, it's all Yin–Yang.' Precisely because Yin–Yang is felt to have universal application, it is vital to study its application in a particular sphere. Only then can the dry concepts Yin and Yang begin to become appreciable and, more importantly, capable of being applied by students.

Taijiquan forms are movements

In Taijiquan it is commonly thought that the names of the postures are for the completed positions so often shown in photographs. This is not strictly accurate. The final posture is like the ripple left on the beach by a wave. It is an echo or reminder of the flow of energy, inertia, Qi, leading to that posture from the previous one. The traditional name refers to the movement flow, *not* to the residual posture left at the end. Each of these flows is described as having a Yin phase or component and a Yang complement. This aspect is the most difficult to express in a book. A book is, after all, a static record of a flow of words. What we are discussing is a flow of movement, not words.

Benefits of Yin–Yang Form study

This aspect of study can be most rewarding and stimulating. We have to try to understand two things simultaneously. These are both the application of the ideas of Yin and Yang to the execution of the moves, and increasingly coming to understand the richness and utility of the concepts themselves. On the one hand, we need to understand why, for example, one part of Brush Knee Push Step is called Yin and another part called Yang, or why some postures are complete with a single Yin–Yang pair (e.g. Brush Knee Push Step), while others can contain several (e.g. Single Whip).

This is to teach us about the postures in the form, the individual waves, segments or elements within the overall flow of a linked round of postures. This helps us to further refine and learn more precisely the execution of moves.

On the other hand, puzzling out why one set of movements is called Yin and another is called Yang forces us to learn the meaning of Yin and Yang. We ask ourselves, 'What have all the Yins got in common? What have all the Yangs got in common?' This gives us both an insight into Chinese philosophy and the opportunity of beginning to apply these categories in our own experience. We very rapidly realise that the greeting card approximation of Yin and Yang, that many people are aware of, is hopelessly naive and contaminated with our cultural ideas and prejudices.

Master Chu liked to recite the following traditional tag: 'Yang is forwards, upwards and outwards. Yin is downwards, inwards and backwards.' There is a great deal more to the Yin–Yang study of forms than just this tag, but it is a useful summary of the main aspects of the Yin–Yang analysis of a movement. Other tags fill out the richness of the concepts of Yin and Yang.

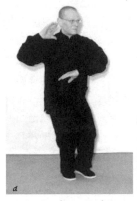
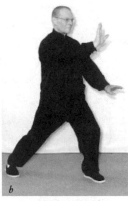
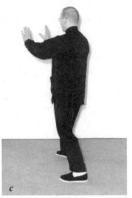

a

b

c

Yin – Brush Knee Push Step

Yang – Brush Knee Push Step, NB phases = 1 move

Entering Single Whip from Yang An

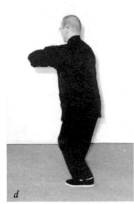
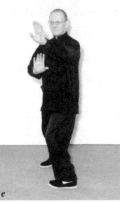
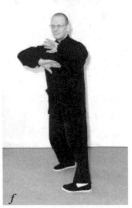

d

e

f

Yin – Single Whip 1st phase

Yang – Single Whip 1st phase

Yin – Single Whip 2nd phase

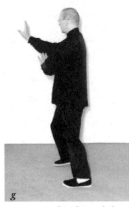
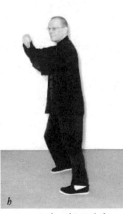
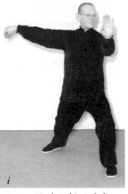

g

h

i

Yang – Single Whip 2nd phase

Yin – Single Whip 3rd phase

Yang – Single Whip 3rd phase: Completion, NB 3 phases = 1 move

'Yang expands/inflates. Yin contracts/deflates/shrinks.'

'Yang is simple and direct. Yin is neither simple nor direct (Yin is complex and subtle).'

'Yang expresses. Yin supports/nurtures.'

As our appreciation of Yin–Yang develops, we can find Yin–Yang aspects of everything in the art. This often acts as a corrective to our prejudices. Particularly in the climate of the current debate about gender, sex roles and stereotyping, a study of a traditional Yin–Yang analysis can be most stimulating and enlightening.

Problems in Yin–Yang Form study

A major problem in attempting to approach Yin–Yang theory is the tendency to equate the translations of Yin – female, woman – and Yang – male, man – with our cultural views of men and women, masculinity and femininity. In our culture we tend to equate female with weak and male with strong. This is instantly in opposition to the Chinese view, where both are equally potent but in qualitatively different and complementary ways. Yin is always the equal and the complement of Yang. Another problem is the little English word 'is'. We see lists of things that are Yin or Yang and tend to read them as 'Yin is dark, soft, female, etc. Yang is bright, hard, male, etc.' In common usage the 'is' relation tends to indicate reciprocity. For example: If A 'is' B, then B 'is' A. So many people slip into the error of thinking that if bright, hard, male, etc. are Yang then Yang must be bright, hard and male. Similarly, if soft, dark, female are Yin then Yin must be soft, dark and female. Unsurprisingly many people become very confused at this point and dismiss the Chinese ideas of Yin and Yang as nonsensical.

Consider these statements:

Ford Mondeo is a car. (Cf. Dark is Yin.)

Honda Civic is a car. (Cf. Soft is Yin.)

Renault Clio is a car. (Cf. Female is Yin.)

Few of us would then say 'A car is Ford Mondeo, Honda Civic, Renault Clio', and then dismiss the idea 'car' as nonsensical. We would probably summarise the original three statements something along the lines of: the Ford Mondeo, Honda Civic and Renault Clio are all cars. More formally the three original statements are taken to indicate the existence of a class, group or set called 'car' of which all three are members. Similarly Yin and Yang are classes.

Yin	Yang
Soft	Hard
Dark	Bright
Female	Male

Using the car example as a model, we can say: soft, dark and female are all Yins. Hard, bright and male are all Yangs. So Yin itself is not soft, dark or female. Yin is Yin. The particular attributes or characteristics *belong* to the class, set or group: Yin. Neither is Yang, itself, hard, bright or male. Yang is Yang. These particular attributes or characteristics *belong* to the class, set or group: Yang.

I see a similarity here with the use of 'x' and 'y' in an equation. The convention is that 'x' stands for 'any number' and 'y' also stands for 'any number'. A particular equation specifies a relationship between 'x' and 'y' such that for a given value of 'x' the value of 'y' can also be stated. Western science and technology has flourished on the basis of the practical usefulness of this level of abstraction. Similarly Yin–Yang theory is the abstraction that underpins Chinese science and technology. If you like, Yin–Yang theory is the 'algebra' and 'calculus' of Chinese thought. The difference being that the Western abstractions 'x' and 'y' are *quantitative* (any number) while the Chinese abstractions are *qualitative* (any attribute or characteristic).

The first step in the application of Yin–Yang to the moves of the form is to mark the points in the flow of the sequence where Yin ends and Yang begins. Also of course the reciprocal points where Yang ends and Yin begins. Fu Zhongwen in his book *Mastering Yang Style Taijiquan* calls these 'Ding Dian'. Literally this would translate as 'fixed point'. Louis Swain in his translation uses the phrase 'the culminating point or ending posture' (Swain 1999).

For some people this immediately creates a problem and causes confusion. How can there be 'fixed points' or 'ending postures' in Taijiquan? Surely one of the things that distinguishes this art is its continuity, its flow? Consider again the waves on the sea, their peaks and troughs. Each peak has a definite top, before falling into the next trough, and each trough a clear bottom before rising again to the next peak. Are these not 'fixed points' or 'culminating points'?

I'd like to draw on mathematics again to clarify this point. I borrow an idea from calculus. This is the branch of mathematics that studies curves and the rate of change of the slopes of curves. A simple waveform is the sine wave.

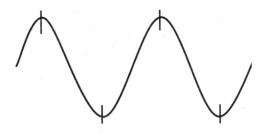

Sine wave showing zero points of inflection

This is a repeating set of curves that rise to a peak and then fall to a trough; over and over again. The rate of change of the curve rises to the peak, slows and eventually reaches zero at the very top. Similarly the rate of change accelerates down towards the bottom of the trough; as the trough is approached the rate slows and finally becomes zero again at the bottom of the trough. These zero points, the top of a peak and the bottom of a trough, are called 'points of inflection'. They are fixed points in the flow of the wave where, however fleetingly, there is a pause before reversing, either from rising to falling or vice versa. This idea of a pause before reversing seems to be implicit in traditional Yin–Yang theory. *The Great Commentary* (*Da Chuan*) of the *I Ching* (*Book of Changes*) discusses the ways of change. One way specified is 'reversal'.

So applying Yin–Yang analysis to the performance of the form in Taijiquan specifies the 'points of inflection' in the flowing wave of the continuous movements: the peaks of Yang and the troughs of Yin. In this sense these are 'fixed points' in the ongoing flow, 'culminating points' or the 'ending postures' at the end of either a Yin phase or a Yang phase.

The Chinese draw an analogy with their writing system here. Chinese characters are built up from individual brush strokes, or lines. A beginner learns to paint each character stroke by stroke. This can be seen as similar to the Western style of writing letters known as printing. When I was a child in primary school this was my first introduction to writing. Later on I was introduced to 'joined up' writing, which is more formally described as cursive script. The Chinese also have a 'joined up' or cursive style of character formation. In this style, rather than building up a character stroke by stroke, the ideal is to write each character with a single flowing move of the brush.

When a student begins to learn Taijiquan the moves are broken down into the equivalent of individual strokes, frequently based on the shift of weight from one foot to the other and the consequential movements of the hands and arms. This allows a given move to be broken down into a number of steps. For example, the first step out, with the right foot, from the initial feet-together starting posture might be broken down into:

1. Empty the right leg (in preparation for the step) by sinking all your weight to your left leg. As you do this, notice how this 'springs' the arms, curved out from the body.

2. Lift the right leg, maintaining knee to elbow connection.

3. Step the right leg out to the right, placing the heel down first.

4. Settle the weight back onto both feet to achieve 'central equilibrium' (both feet equally share the body's weight). Notice as you do this how the wrists bend as the ankles take the body's weight.

This is the first move, or 'Shi' in Chinese. It can be viewed as a 'four stroke' move analogous to a character composed of four strokes. Executing the move in this step-wise or individual 'stroke' fashion may be seen as 'printing' the move. However, all these individual moves combine to form a single step. So pursuing the writing analogy these individual moves must be 'joined up' as the single strokes of a 'printed' character are joined up to create the 'cursive' form of that single character. In terms of Yin–Yang analysis this move is a single Yin or Yang phase. This specific, initial, step is Yin.

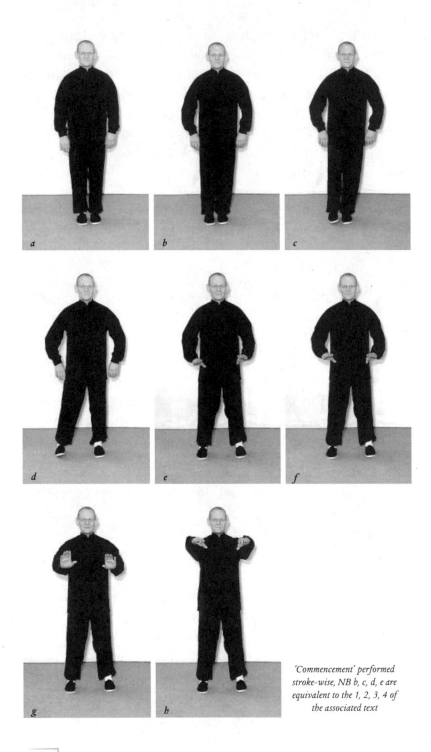

'Commencement' performed stroke-wise, NB b, c, d, e are equivalent to the 1, 2, 3, 4 of the associated text

It is a gathering and preparation prior to the expressing of the arms forward and upwards. In this sense it is the 'mother' of the following move. Part of the traditional definition of Yin is the phrase 'Yin is the Mother of Yang'. The end of the step is the end point, the 'Ding Dian' in Fu Zhongwen's terminology, a 'culminating point' or 'ending posture' in Swain's translation (Swain 1999), or a 'point of inflection' in my mathematical analogy.

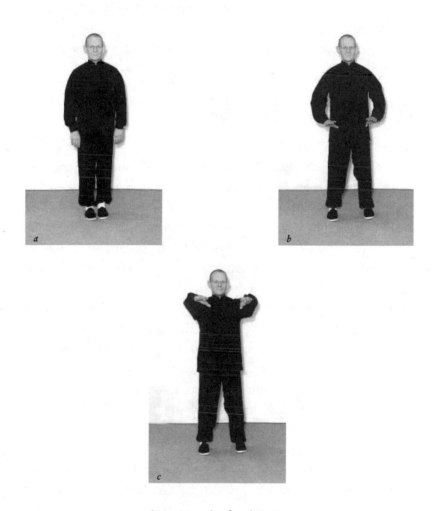

'Commencement' performed Yin–Yang

The initial stroke-wise method of execution can be a little clunky and appear rather robotic. The 'joined up' style derived from the Yin–Yang analysis reveals the rhythm and flow of the form, what Chen Man Ch'ing referred to as the 'swing and sway' of the form. Without this insight the 'printed' stroke-wise execution of the form either results in robo Taijiquan or, in the pursuit of flow, the form degenerates into a sloppy spaghetti style that is vague and incoherent. This Yin–Yang analysis is similar to the Fourier analysis of a complex waveform into a series of simpler waves, which when combined result in a waveform of the same shape as the original.

Stages of Yin–Yang study

There are two stages, or phases, in the Yin–Yang Form study. The first stage is primarily the responsibility of the teacher. Students must be able to perform the round of the form by themselves and so be familiar with the raw outline of their form before they can be able to study the 'joined up', or cursive, Yin–Yang version. Having led the student to this level of accomplishment, the teacher now must help point out the 'Ding Dian', or 'points of inflection'. This is initially a form of 'punctuating' the form and may seem somewhat arbitrary to some students. As the form is being performed the teacher may start by 'singing' the Yin and Yang phases to mark the 'Ding Dian', points of inflection.

Then the form may be reviewed, move-by-move, posture-by-posture, to indicate that a particular string of movement, frequently associated with stepping or shifting the weight, is either Yin or Yang. Here the teacher will demonstrate more of the internal characteristics of the string, be it Yin or Yang, using tag descriptions/definitions of Yin and Yang.

For example, the teacher may abstract a segment from the form saying something like: From *here* to *here* is Yin, or Yang, as the case may be. Then, using the traditional tag formulae, the teacher will show how this abstracted segment of the form conforms to either the Yin aspect or the Yang aspect of the tag. Saying something like: Yin shrinks, contracts, deflates, condenses and hence can be seen as moving in an inward direction in all three dimensions – 'Yin is inward, downward and backward' as Master Chu would say. See how my body and my limbs move in this way during this chunk. Now you practise this piece and try to feel that you do it in such a way that you too move 'downward, inwards, backward', condensing, deflating and contracting as you go.

When the students can demonstrate some competence, at least starting and stopping in the right place, and also some competence at moving in the broadly appropriate fashion, expanding or contracting, inflating or shrinking, then the teacher can move on to the next chunk, be it Yin or Yang.

One important tag to consider is: 'Yang is simple and direct. Yin is neither simple nor direct (Yin is complex and subtle).' A general characteristic of Yang phase movement segments is that they are 'simple and direct'. You should be able to feel, and express, this relatively easily. For example, the move 'An', frequently translated as 'Push', is Yang, and a pretty basic and clear Yang at that. As is the concluding Yang phase of the move 'Lou Xi Ao Bu', 'Brush Knee Push Step'. They both should feel similar as you execute them.

Yin moves, by contrast, are neither simple nor direct. Typically Yin phase segments are more articulated than Yang phase segments. Going back to the ideograph analogy, Yin phase moves will be built up from more strokes than Yang phase moves.

This process of teacher teaching/demonstrating and student practising, learning and studying is repeated until

Yin–Yang comparison

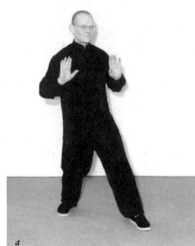

Yin – An

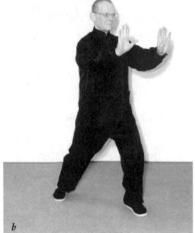

Yang – An

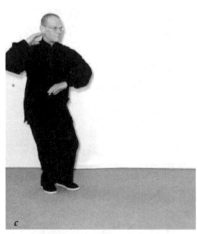

Yin – Brush Knee Push Step

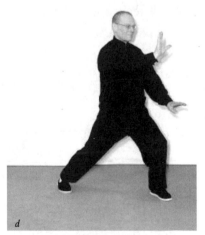

Yang – Brush Knee Push Step

the entire form has been covered. The students should now at least be aware of the 'Ding Dian' points along the way throughout the form. This could be considered the end of the first phase of Yin–Yang Form study.

The second stage is much more the responsibility of the individual student. Equipped with the information and demonstrations of the teacher, the students now must find and cultivate these Yin–Yang features and attributes in their own performance. It is the student's personal responsibility to realise the teacher's teaching in practice. This is a typically Chinese attitude. I remember a teacher in Taipei, Taiwan, who expressed himself most bluntly. On accepting me as a student he said, 'OK. I teach. You practise.'

Two other teachers independently stressed the importance of the student's participation in the active learning necessary for any real accomplishment. They both stressed that a student should *never* take anything a teacher said simply on trust. Anything you get from a teacher is only a working hypothesis until you can realise it in practice.

In this, and all the subsequent forms of the Six Secrets, you, the student, do *not* simply rote learn the relevant words. You learn to 'sing the songs' of the individual secrets by learning to simply report your immediate experiences of each particular element. This is not very different from the advanced driving exercise where the driver maintains a running commentary on the road conditions, signs, other vehicles and pedestrians. In the use of the Six Secrets as an aid to development in Taijiquan the commentary is restricted to a single feature at a time. It is as if the driver were to only report road conditions, or other vehicles or pedestrians, on any given drive.

So now the truth of the assertion that the whole form is only Yin–Yang becomes clear. It is a continuously changing flow of complex movements, expressing multiple instances of the concepts Yin and Yang. It becomes a movement poem, a paean of Yin–Yang expressed in movement. This can very appropriately become one of several possible meditations in performing Taijiquan or Qi Gong forms.

3. 'SPIRAL', OR QI, FORM

After Yin–Yang, which analyses the form into its natural elements and components, the remaining secrets are concerned with refining the details of the expression and execution of those elements. This is increasingly subtle Daoyin.

In Yin–Yang study the emphasis is on the core facet of expansion–contraction, or, if you prefer, grow–shrink or inflate–deflate. Your limbs move relative to your body either, in Master Chu's tag, forward, upward, outward – Yang – or backward, downward, inward – Yin. In Spiral Form the impact of *movement* of the body in space in terms of stepping and rotating is additionally considered.

From standing practice, Jing Gong, the gentle, fundamental, core movement of the natural work of the body, is appreciated. This can be considered the *Qi of breathing*, or more precisely the Qi that is in the breath. Relative to the body the limbs either move towards the torso in a contracting, or deflating, fashion or they move away from the torso in an expanding, or inflating, fashion. The former is called 'He' in Chinese, the latter 'Kai'. In English, 'Kai' and 'He' are frequently translated as 'open/opening' and 'close/closing'.

The elbows, and their movements, are now the primary focus of study. Again it must be emphasised that without familiarity with both the sequence of the moves of the form and their 'punctuation', provided from Yin–Yang study, this emphasis on the elbows can easily be counterproductive. The ball and socket joint of the shoulder needs to be very loose and mobile to ensure full rotational articulation so that the elbows can 'flap' easily. To achieve this necessary shoulder looseness and relaxation the many hours of practice of initial form learning and Yin–Yang Form study are essential. This initial degree of shoulder loosening can be greatly enhanced by Spiral Form study.

The major new technical terms now are 'Kai' and 'He', 'open' and 'close' in English. When the distance between the torso and the arm, as measured by the movement and position of the elbow, increases this is called 'Kai' or 'open'. It might be more useful to say in English 'opening' to stress the dynamic nature of this feature. Conversely when the distance decreases this is called 'He' or 'close'. Again 'closing' may be a more useful English translation.

One important thing to remember during form study is that, unlike the static feet of Jing Gong practice, in form the feet move. Standing practice is the Yin cultivating, nurturing, preparing side of the art of Taijiquan and as such can be called 'Movement in stillness', that is mostly Yin (still) with a dot of Yang (moving) within.

Any other practice is the Yang expressing, developing and performing/executing side of the art and as such can be called 'stillness in movement'. Symbolically this is the other 'fish' in the 'Two Fish' Yin–Yang diagram – Taiji Tu. It is mostly Yang (moving) with a dot of Yin (stillness).

This movement of the feet, and hence of the entire body, introduces a new subtlety to the terms 'Kai' and 'He'. The distance between the elbow and the torso may be affected by the movement of the torso as much as by the movement of the arm. The arm may move relative to the torso. The

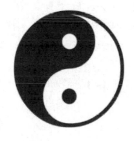

Taiji Tu diagram

torso may move relative to the arm. Both arm and torso may move simultaneously, either in the same or different directions. Thus unlike static practice when both arms will move in the same fashion, either opening 'Kai', or both closing 'He', in moving practices one arm may be opening while the other is closing.

The use of the terms 'Kai' and 'He' simplifies this complexity by focusing on the outcome as measured by the distance from the elbow to the torso. Regardless of the particular elements of a change in this distance, it is the degree and direction of change that is important. If the distance between the torso and the elbow reduces it is called 'He'. Conversely if that distance increases it is called 'Kai'. These changes are always characterised by a rotation around the central axis of the arms, spiralling, the 'flapping' of the elbows.

Perhaps an illustration would be useful here. Consider the first, forward single Peng (Ward Off) in the form. First you sink into your left leg, rotate to the right, and transfer your weight to the right leg holding a ball over the right foot with the right hand on top – the Yin phase; then you step forward with your left leg, transfer the weight forward and expand both arms, the left arm finishing curved with the palm in front of your face – the Yang phase.

Without the rotation, in any Yin phase the arms both shrink towards the torso. However, in this particular example there is a rotation to the right. This rotation moves the torso towards the right arm and away from the left arm; as a consequence of the rotation the distance between the right arm and the torso is reduced while the distance between the torso and the left arm is increased. The right arm, 'He', closes; while the left arm, 'Kai', opens.

In the following Yang phase, the weight shifts forward. The torso moves away from the right hand – the right arm 'Kai' opens. Since it is in the nature of Yang to expand or inflate the arms away from the torso, the left arm also 'Kai' opens.

So now the qualitative description of this first Peng initially classifies it into a subset of moves comprising the Yin phase and another subset of moves comprising the Yang phase. To this description the Spiral Form analysis adds the details of the arm movements classifying them as either Kai, opening, or He, closing. Specifically, in the Yin phase the right arm is He, closing, while the left arm is Kai, opening, and in the Yang phase both arms Kai, open.

Straight away we can see that Kai may appear in both a Yin and a Yang variety. Further analysis reveals that He may also appear in both Yin and Yang varieties. Good examples of Yang He can be found in, for example, An – Push, or Lou Xi Ao Bu – Brush Knee Push Step (see photo series on p.170).

An arm spiral, Kai, open/opening, or He, close/closing, is a local description of the arm–torso distance, measured at the elbow. Yin–Yang is a more global description of a group of body movements. A single posture, say Peng – Ward Off, is made of many individual sub-moves and shifts of weight. These are globally grouped into two sets, the Yin set and the Yang set, which I am calling the Yin phase and the Yang phase. Thus any given Kai or He may occur as part of a Yin phase or Yang phase. The phase determines the quality of the particular opening or closing spiral. The Yang phase opens, expands or inflates globally, hence both Yang Kai (opening) and Yang He (closing) are felt or experienced as spiralling forward, upward and outward. Similarly in any Yin phase both the Kai (opening) and He (closing) are felt or experienced as spiralling backward, downward and inward.

To teach this facet the teacher may again 'sing the Song of Spiral' as the form is performed, specifying, 'Right arm opening, left closing. Both opening, both closing, etc.' Much more useful is detailed demonstration and student practice of moves. Since 'moves' are now 'sets', the Yin phase set and the Yang phase set, Yin–Yang Form study is a necessary prerequisite to Spiral Form study. Again, as always, the responsibility rests with each individual student to realise the information from the teacher. First the student must *find* their own unique and personal 'spirals' in their form. We must relax – 'Fang Song' – to discover the spirals that the body 'wants' to express. Then we must work to remove all obstacles to their fluid and free expression. Finally we, too, will be able to 'sing the Song of Spiral' – not by rote, but simply reporting what we feel is occurring as we perform the form. Thus the whole process becomes an exercise in expanding awareness.

Spiral Form study begins the study of the *Qi of movement*, or more precisely the Qi that is in movement. The formal definitions of Qi contain the following tags, or formulae:

Qi is in movement but it is not movement.

Qi is in breathing but it is not breath.

Earlier I described the movements of a Rectified body, the preferred, most likely or spontaneous movements, as the tracks, or spoor, of Qi. These can be grouped into two sets. The first set is the set of moves observed when the feet remain fixed. The second set is the set of moves observed when the feet move and step with consequent shifts of weight. The first set is primarily the consequence of breathing and so reveal the *Qi of breathing*, though this is shorthand for the more precise 'Qi that is in the breath but not breath itself'. The second set is the consequence of moving the feet, stepping and the consequent shifting of weight; these reveal the *Qi of moving*, which is again shorthand for 'Qi that is in movement but not movement itself'.

The art of Taijiquan aims to develop and use Qi – the Qi that is in both moving and breathing but is *itself* neither breathing nor moving. In order to do this successfully both

Yin Qi and Yang Qi must be found, examined and developed for use. Yin Qi can be related to the Qi of breathing and may be studied through the Yin practices of 'movement in stillness'. Yang Qi can be related to the Qi of moving and may be studied through the Yang practices of 'stillness in movement'. Specifically, increasingly detailed analysis and practice of the Daoyin of the moves of the form through the last four of the Six Secrets is now the path to further accomplishment.

Spiral Form studies the rotational component of the movements of the body and its parts, hence spiral. The exercise to learn Daoyin, which I described in Chapter 6, can also be used to study this opening and closing in the elbows. Since the elbow is the middle joint of the arm, if it moves so does the whole arm. The arm rotates along its length. From learning 'Spiral in the arm', it is the student's responsibility to spread this feeling throughout the whole body. The later secrets both allow and encourage this spreading out.

Problems in Spiral Form study

In the testing required to study and develop Spiral Form students frequently have their initial experience of moving, or bouncing away, their partners. This is partly a result of the change in style of testing now required. In Chapter 3 I discussed the Three Levels of Testing. I called them *Static testing*, *Moving testing* and *Dynamic testing*. The testing primarily used during the initial Rectification of the body is simple Static testing. The student adopts a particular posture and relaxes into it. A tester applies pressure in the appropriate fashion for that particular posture to test the degree to which the student is manifesting a Rectified body. Since now the focus of study is movement, the testing must similarly change from Static to Moving.

In Moving testing the tester still applies appropriate pressure but the student must move slowly and gently to see the effect on both the tester and the student's own body and felt sense of degree of muscular effort. A successful test of this type results in the tester being moved while both the tester and the student agree that the degree of effort on the student's part is reduced to a minimum.

For example, the first forward Peng is often tested (Moving testing) by having the student complete the Yin phase and pausing while the tester places one hand on the student's left elbow and the other on the student's left wrist. The student executes the Yang phase while focusing particularly on the opening Spirals in both arms. Since the tester's job is just to act as a sort of amplifier for the student's sensations, the tester remains relatively passive, simply providing a source of constant pressure.

The experience of the development of this facet can deeply impress the student. Study seems to be definitely bearing fruit. This experience of the Spirals gives sensations that can lead us to imagine we are sensing an energy flow. The mysterious Qi seems to be coming through at last, hence the alternative name of Qi form. However, it is a mistake to regard this level as the pinnacle of practice and achievement. To the extent that this level can be called a Qi form, it is only a pseudo Qi. There is considerable further development possible. The final goal is to achieve a condition where the mind leads the Qi. The Qi leads the body.

At the moment our study of the experience of the natural movements to be found in the Rectified, moving body is still relatively external. I have already called these natural moves, however subtle, the spoor or tracks of Qi. This approach to study examines and explores these mechanical moves and sensations to provide 'directions of intent' that the Yi can ultimately use to direct Qi, and hence the body and its movements, directly. Practising the form exercises and develops the body so that it is capable of clearly and freely expressing the moves and techniques to be found in the form. Practising must also refine and clarify the sensations that accompany moving. These sensations train the 'directions of intent' that the Yi will subsequently use to move the body through moving the Qi. Eventually you no longer think of the move as a name, or even a pattern of movements – however organised and refined. You simply think of the felt sense of the move and, presto, the move has been made in all its subtlety, refinement and power. This is genuinely internal practice: the Gong Fu of Nei Gong training. To get there further work must be undertaken.

The Six Secrets have three remaining topics. These are physical refinements that precede, in a traditional sense, true Nei Gong – 'inner work' or 'internal breathing'. To really be able to talk about Qi, those further physical 'gates' must be passed, or at least well investigated. Qi proper is the topic of the final and infinite study of Nei Gong. As the Taijiquan classics say: 'At first you must be guided through the gate and shown the Way. Afterwards you are free and can go your own way.'

We must be on our guard not to get stuck at a particular level of achievement, nor should we become attached to any particular concept, no matter how powerful it might seem. Strictly speaking the Qi of the Spiral or 'Qi' Form is still external. It relies on the mechanics of the movements, and their interrelationships with the body parts. With its emphasis on spirals and rotation, it tends to focus the attention on the movements of the skin and the body surface.

This cannot yet be really internal, despite both the sophistication of movement that it requires and demonstrates, and the power that can reside in this form of movement. The concentration and focus required at this level is a very profound concentration meditation. However, we must never forget that our method is always Daoyin. Never impose spiral movement as this would lead to too much stiffness and tension in the arms. It can also lead to too much mental activity. If you find a tendency to sweat excessively from the scalp and your hair gets very sweaty, then you are probably over-concentrating. This indicates too much Yi (will) and not enough Xin (feeling) or, if you like, too much 'inducing' without sufficient attention to finding the 'guide'. I have a tendency in this direction myself, so I know what I'm talking about.

4. CENTRE-TURN FORM

Perhaps the most frequently referred-to level, when considering the details of performance, is the Centre-Turn Form. It is not always as well understood as it might be. The centre can be visualised as a point, rather like the initial grain of sand around which a pearl grows. It is found to be the point of intersection between Zhong Mai, the central channel between Ni Wan and Hui Yin, and the horizontal line joining Qi Hai and Ming Men in the Rectified body. The Qi sinks to the centre and coalesces, or accumulates, around it. This can be at first imagined and then experienced as a ball or sphere inside the pelvis. This is the meaning of the term 'Dantien' in Taijiquan.

It is important to realise that the Qi forms a *sphere*, or *ball*, around the centre. This is a vital visualisation and an eventual accomplishment. Your centre is a point. A point is dimensionless. It has no length, breadth or depth. It has no surface. Without a surface, the points of which can rotate, 'turning' is impossible. However, if you visualise a ball of Qi centred on your centre, you can express this physically and can roll, or turn, this sphere of Qi. You can learn to move your Dantien. Like the so-called Qi in the 'Qi' or Spiral Form being pseudo Qi, the centre of the Centre-Turn Form is an approximation, or pseudo centre.

To talk about Centre-Turns is a convenient verbal shorthand. The centre, in this sense, can move forwards and backwards, right and left, up and down. The sphere of Qi rotates on one of the three Cartesian axes (see the figure opposite).

In the art of Taijiquan the rotation of the Dantien (centre) around the vertical axis is particularly relevant. As long as we maintain vertical posture with both feet on the ground the vertical axis is primary. Since this is the case, throughout the execution of the form it may be more useful to talk about *central* turning much of the time. This direction of turning affects the rotation of the torso in the hip sockets, the centre of the region called 'Kua' in Chinese.

Centre-Turn Form is particularly interested in the relationship between the torso and the legs. The torso may move from being balanced on one leg to being balanced on the other. The torso may rotate relative to a given leg or a leg may rotate relative to the torso.

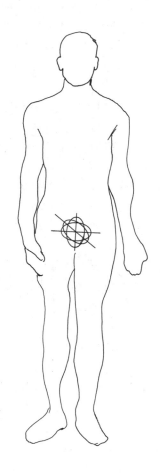

Lower Dantien

First let us consider shifting the weight from one leg to the other. In Taijiquan the most important shift of weight is that from the back leg to the front leg in a basic front stance, sometimes called a 'Mountain climbing step' or more generically in Wu Shu 'Gong Bu'.

181

Because of the nature of the hip/leg joint – a ball-like lump on the top of the femur (upper leg bone) and the acetabulum (the rounded pocket in the pelvis that accepts the ball of the femur) – whenever we completely relax into a single leg for support there is a small rotational settle towards the supporting leg. Without this it is impossible to fully 'empty' the other leg such that it is instantly ready to move. Thus in any shift of leg to either left or right there is also a rotation to either left or right. This means that the sphere of the Dantien will also rotate either left or right. Since the tube of the erect torso sits on this sphere it too will rotate. This is Centre-Turn producing *central* turning of the torso.

In the transfer of the weight of the basic front stance the width of the stance must also be considered. In Taijiquan the feet are commonly maintained 'shoulder width' apart. This means that a straightforward shift of weight is not in fact 'straight' in the sense of directly forward. In moving the body forward the lateral, sideways, component cannot fail to have an impact. Thus the central channel, Zhong Mai, of the torso does not move straightforward but on a diagonal vector, leftward or rightward depending on which foot is in front, left or right.

Since the shift of weight starts and finishes 'single weighted' there must also be, however small, a rotation of the centre and consequent central rotation of the torso. The conventional description of the centre movement in this forward shift of weight is 'forward *and* left' (or right as the case may be).

There are of course many other possibilities to explore and add to our increasing repertoire of sensations of the subtleties of the body's movements. These sensations further develop and refine our felt picture of the move and so form the increasingly detailed 'directions of intent' that the Yi uses to directly affect the Qi flows and hence the moving of the body. The centre may move the torso. It may also 'pull' or 'push' the Kua and so effect the movement of the legs, turning them either towards or away from the torso, which will also be rotating either toward or away from the leg in question. This 'pulling' and 'pushing' of the Kua may also be described, perhaps somewhat confusingly, as He and Kai of the Kua. That is Kua 'closing' or 'opening'.

The teacher will again illustrate and demonstrate these moves while the students practise and repeat them. Once more the teacher may 'sing' the Centre-Turns as part or all of the form is performed. Again the students will develop the ability to sing along simply by reporting their increasing awareness of the movements of the centre.

The three Cartesian axes, or Three Circles, may be labelled 'x' for the vertical axis (the flat circle), 'y' for the horizontal axis (the front circle) and 'z' for the forward–backward axis (the side circle).

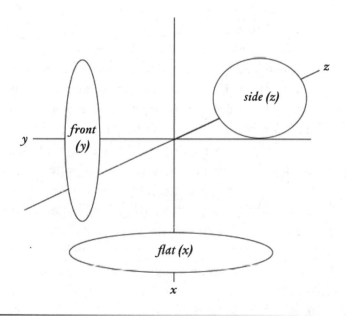

Three Cartesian axes, x, y, z, showing Three Circles: x = flat circle, y = front circle, z = side circle

Rotation around the 'x' axis will turn the centre, and hence the torso, left and right. Rotation around the 'y' axis will roll the sphere of the Dantien either forward/down or backward/up. Rotation around the 'z' axis will bring the feet over the head in a sideways cartwheel either clockwise or anti-clockwise. This last direction of centre movement becomes much more relevant in situations where you are no longer standing on your feet, such as wrestling or ground fighting. Since this book only attempts to provide a sketch of the stages in accomplishing the art of Taijiquan, I shall leave further elaboration and detail to your own practice.

Centre-Turns of the Qi ball can be executed apart from spirals. The testing of the Centre-Turn again bounces the partner away but there is a different quality about the effect. It is realised that the rotations of the centre are, in fact, the spiral movement of the centre. With this realisation, the centre move, as a spiral, can serve as the genesis movement of the spirals of the Spiral Form.

I would like to emphasise that all this talk of circles and spirals ultimately is only a way of talking about concrete experiences of movement. Rarely do movements use more than a section, or a chord for the geometers amongst you, of any circle so do not go looking to perform 360-degree full circles. There is a real risk that some readers may *think* they have grasped the use of the Three-Circle concept when all they have in fact is an intellectual, not experiential, understanding. Some of you will grasp this concept easily. Indeed you may already have. Others may find that the idea is going straight over your heads. In which case there is no need for concern, simply wait until your experience matches the idea. I recommend that if it is not immediately clear to you so that you can incorporate it into your performance that you ask your teacher to demonstrate and explain.

The two forms, Yin–Yang and spiral, then merge into each other. This adds a considerable depth to the movements of the form. It can be regarded as deep Daoyin, relative to the earlier attempts to find the Dao (Tao) of the movements of the body. It is a level of practice that indicates that considerable success has been achieved in the Rectification of the body. A Taijiquan player who can achieve both the merger of Yin–Yang and Spiral forms and integrate this merged form with the Centre-Turn form is well accomplished and has a very solid foundation for Qi development and inner cultivation. Through the use of the Xin to inform the Yi our practice now develops a good repertoire of 'directions of intent' to drive the execution of the form by 'mind alone'. The study of the Centre-Turn Form can only be pursued effectively through the use of the Xin – your sensitivity. Generally attempts to 'make' the turns of the Dantien result in excessively large movements that result in the disruption of the integrity of the Rectified body. The genuine movements of the Dantien are very small. The Yi must be restrained to only offer 'directions of intent' for the moving centre. Most attempts to deliberately move the centre will be, at least initially, far too gross to be correct, beneficial or effective.

This will be revealed in the Moving testing of the Centre-Turn aspects of each move. The more the student *tries* to move the tester by Centre-Turn alone the less effective the student is likely to be. Only when the student can learn the trick of simply relaxing and ensuring that the required 'direction of intent' is clearly expressed will the tester be effortlessly bounced off. This is not at all easy. However, when it is, however erratically and fleetingly, initially experienced, the truth of the tag 'less is more' becomes apparent.

The pairing of Spiral and Centre-Turn forms is analogous to the two levels that emerged from the Yin–Yang study. The conclusion there was that the Taijiquan form is all Yin–Yang, due to the Yin–Yang components of every form, the individual forms being the level above Yin–Yang and, in a sense, derived from it. Similarly, the spiralling of the centre is the source from which the spirals of the Spiral Form are the expression. It is also the source of the next Secret: Spiral in the leg.

5. SPIRAL IN THE LEG

This level of practice is often neglected. Put into words, it sounds very simple. It applies the concepts from the previous two topics to the legs. The leg spiral is always Kai, 'opening', in Taijiquan. This helps to develop strong roots. However, ,we must not forget that Kai may come in either a Yin or Yang flavour. Thus while the leg spiral is always Kai, which particular flavour of Kai, Yin or Yang, will be a function of the Yin–Yang phase appropriate at that particular moment. Every movement, and shift of weight, should 'open' the knees slightly. When you shift your weight into a leg, that leg 'opens'. The emptying of the leg from which the weight is coming must not cause the empty leg to collapse or 'close'.

Not collapsing the knees is part of Three Circle Theory, but this can be a bit stiff or rigid. Spiral in the legs, open spiral, can help to make the legs less stiff. When the legs are moved to the side, or round the body, leading with the knees can help stability. The kicks, Separate Left, Separate Right and Lotus Kick, become much easier and more understand-able using open spiral in the legs, leading with the knees. They are revealed as 'Peng' in the legs and become the leg equivalent of the posture 'Slant Flying' in the arms.

Again it must be emphasised that leg spirals are tiny. Attempts to make or do leg spirals are doomed to failure. Leg spirals are best effected through clear use of the Yi to empha-sise the appropriate 'direction of intent'.

Separate Kick as 'Peng'

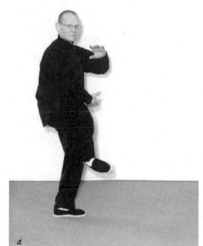

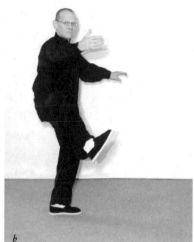

Yin – Leg 'Peng'

Yang – Leg 'Peng'

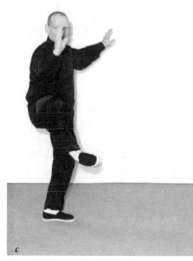

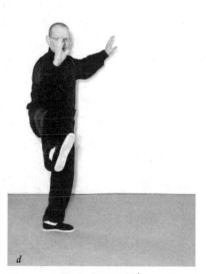

Yin – Separate Kick

Yang – Separate Kick

Finally, to really understand the action of the centre to pull and push the limbs, spiral in the legs cannot be neglected. This study helps to connect the Qi from the heels, through the centre, into the torso, upper limbs and head. Some people maintain that it is best studied and developed in Pushing Hands practice. Even so, it is a worthwhile focus for form practice, especially for those who either do not, or cannot, practise pushing hands.

Some readers may feel that my discussion of leg spiral is particularly sketchy and that I have not really explained it. They would be right. I have deliberately kept this description of leg spiral rather slim as messing about with your legs incorrectly can easily produce problems with the knees and ankles. I have given enough hints to assist development for those ready to explore this area. For all others I refer you to your teachers.

6. YIN–YANG HEAD AND HANDS

This is the pinnacle of precision of description and execution of the physical forms of Taijiquan. It is a further refinement of the spiral concept, which started relatively externally in the limbs and became more internal as it moved towards the centre. Simply put (but please do not assume it is simple in practice) this level is concerned with the study of the counter spirals between the sides of the neck and the movements of the hands.

More colloquially this is also sometimes called 'Twisting the dishcloth'. When we wring out a cloth we most commonly turn one hand clockwise and the other anti-clockwise. In this most refined level of physical movement study we examine the relative movements of the pelvis and pectoral girdles – the hips and shoulders. This is a most refined

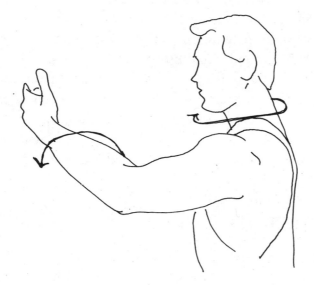

Yin–Yang: Head–Hands

Yin–Yang study. The relative movements are miniscule and must never be forced or imposed. They can only be discovered and cultivated.

This study perfects the description of the physical detail of the movements contained in forms. In experience it will be found that seeking for the neck/palm connection and dynamic refines the perception and execution of the Centre-Turns and hence the spiral component of the forms.

Again I have kept this discussion of Yin–Yang: Head–Hands brief quite deliberately. Without a good foundation in all the preceding five secrets any attempt to pursue Yin–Yang: Head–Hands could be hazardous, not to say counterproductive. Trying to add in refinements willy nilly with no respect for the necessary natural order of progression and refinement would not be a good thing. Either wait until your own practice gives you these higher secrets or wait until your teacher teaches the finer refinements in person so that you can experience and see their physical reality, not just think you have grasped these ideas intellectually. Being able to play properly is more important than mere intellectual achievement.

CONCLUSION

The Three Circle study establishes a foundation and repertoire for an alphabet of movement. The Yin–Yang study develops a qualitative description of the pattern and flow and elements of form. The next four develop the fine grain, the internal structure, of the outwardly visible forms.

Additionally the climbing of the ladder of the Six Secrets increasingly shifts the emphasis from training the Xin to training the Yi. Starting with the Spiral Form the testing, of increasingly subtle and refined movements, reveals the necessity to refrain from doing too much or trying to impose movements on the body. The Yi must be trained to provide clear 'directions of intent' to guide the Natural and intrinsic movements. It must be disciplined to refrain from trying to usurp the body's self-sufficient movement.

The presence of these 'internal' details, not immediately obvious to the untrained eye, explains why some arts, and Taijiquan especially, are referred to as 'half-open door' arts.

By copying a Tai Chi player, most people can learn to produce a dance that resembles a Taijiquan form. But without an understanding of, or training in, the details, they would only have half the art. They would have the rough outline but not the detail or the knowledge of how to develop and refine — polish, if you like — the roughly blocked-in moves.

At the end of the study of all Six Secrets, we have two complementary, detailed descriptions or analyses of Qi developing movement, with qualitative and quantitative detail. We know how the movements should feel and we know precisely what their trajectories, origins and terminations should be. However, all this can still be regarded as external in a certain sense, since however subtle it has become it is still basically mechanical.

None of these details must be taken as instructions. Never try to make these movements happen. We must work to discover these details inherent in our execution of the moves of the form. Once discovered we must nurture, or cultivate, these details so that they grow and develop into full flower. The Chinese have a tag: 'Find. Cultivate/Train. Use.' Through our own practice and the guidance of a good teacher we can 'Find'. Through dedicated and mindful practice we can 'Cultivate' and train what we have found. Finally this work allows use to 'Use' our selves most efficiently and naturally.

A fellow teacher and friend lists the stages of development as follows:

1. Unconsciously incompetent.

2. Consciously incompetent.

3. Consciously competent.

4. Unconsciously competent.

I would map these onto the Chinese tag as follows:

1. Unconsciously incompetent – before we start study.

2. Consciously incompetent – the initial 'Find' stage, re-alising how corrupt and unnatural our movement is and focusing in on natural movement.

3. Consciously competent – the 'Cultivate' stage, working to train and develop our natural movement, 'dredging the channels' as the Chinese would say.

4. Unconsciously competent – the 'Use' stage, when we reap the harvest of all our hard work.

Chapter 8	# Practise to Perfection

THE SYLLABUS OF TAIJIQUAN

I have completed the description of my sketch of the ladder of Six Secrets used by Chu King Hung in his teaching of Taijiquan. My writing about the art has been organised around three ideas, which I regard as three developmental tasks or levels of learning. The first is Rectification of the body, the second is the method, Daoyin, and the third I call Nei Gong, linking the Six Secrets with true Nei Gong of 'internal work' or 'internal breathing'. The Six Secrets are in a sense part of the description of the art of Taijiquan, which makes it a particular, unique 'Quan'.

These levels of learning circle round and round. Rectification develops Daoyin, which further develops both Rectification and Nei Gong. Any part of the cycle can be the starting point, so, however long you practise and study Taijiquan, there will always be something to work on and towards.

I have chosen this structure so as to be able to develop a syllabus that depends less on the externally obvious actions than on the different developmental tasks required. It has a certain parallel with ideas of the 'San Cai', three powers, of Heaven, People and Earth.

- Earth phase = Rectification of the body.

- People phase = Learning, study and practice of Daoyin.

- Heaven phase = Nei Gong, Six Secrets, the physical practice of Taijiquan to link 'Heaven' and 'Earth'.

I have tried to explain that the art of Taijiquan also contains methods, as well as its more obvious techniques. At different stages, different methods, focuses or objectives are appropriate. The same, or apparently the same, techniques can be the object of study, using different methods; for example, any posture can teach, demonstrate or develop different aspects.

The posture Brush Knee Push Step can be practised for Rectification. You can stand still and sink into your image of the posture, or you can repeat the posture in an endless chain, concentrating on hanging from your head, feeling 'Song' in all directions, with your elbows over your knees. It can also be practised for Daoyin, feeling the way the movements of the torso and limbs are following guide paths, almost like tracks in the air. Then the Yin part and the Yang part can be explored, either in their own right, or as part of Daoyin, or as part of one of the other secrets – Spiral, or Centre-Turn, and the rest.

To an inexperienced observer, it appears that everyone is doing the 'same' move, but, to the trained eye, the different methods and levels become clear. Taijiquan is a half-open door art. It has ceased to be an imperial, or aristocratic or clan, treasure hidden from outsiders, so it is no longer a closed-door art. However, particularly for Westerners, the door into Taijiquan is not wide open. Without the grounding in ideas, learned 'at your mother's knee', that a Chinese child soaks up, we can look at the players and still miss details. Yang Lu-Shan may have learnt his art from watching through a crack in the wall at the Chen practice, but he was reckoned to be something of a genius, as well as having the necessary background. The Taijiquan classics clearly state the need for a teacher.

THE TAIJIQUAN TEACHER'S JOB

The teacher's job, in any 'Quan', is to teach both the moves and techniques, and the methods that make up that particular 'Quan'. With any teaching, a certain amount of change in students is both inevitable and expected. For if your practice had no effect you would probably stop trying. However, in Taijiquan the physical moves are only half the story. They are the external, observable consequences of the Qi flow.

Since the teacher aims to assist students in their cultivation of Qi, teaching the moves is only part of the teacher's job, and not necessarily the major part. Helping students to clear out their bodies to remove blockages and wastings is primary. Then helping them to find and develop their Qi in movement – teaching Daoyin – becomes important. This follows the principle: 'Give food to the starving and you feed them today. Teach them to farm and you feed them for the rest of their lives.'

The particular moves and postures of the different schools of Taijiquan are the vehicles chosen by the Masters of those schools, which then become the evidence of students' accomplishment. Differences between schools and styles are frequently differences in emphasis in teaching; what is important and when. For example, Chen style emphasises 'Chansi Jin' or, in my terms, 'Spiral', Yang style is noted for openness or 'Song' with its long open postures, while Wu style lays stress on 'open' and 'closed' Qi and breathing techniques. All three styles overlap each other considerably and, at their zenith, all have 'Chansi Jin', 'Song' and 'opening/closing' of Qi and breathing.

What makes Taijiquan unique is not so much the techniques as such but also the methods of acquisition, development and execution of those techniques. One student of mine was a highly ranked practitioner of ju-jitsu. Others of my students, who were only familiar with my teaching of Taijiquan, were somewhat confused as to why this man felt the need to study with me. His answer is revealing. In essence what he said was that while I did little to him that his other teachers had not done the *way* I did what I did was unique in his experience. *That* was why he wished to study with me. He wanted to understand how he, too, could acquire such seemingly effortless and powerful techniques.

It is this *Way* that I am trying to explain, the Way of: Rectification, Daoyin and Nei Gong. A frequent tag formula that we repeat regularly in my school is 'Find. Train. Use'; often when translating, translators feel the need to insert the pronoun 'it' to conform to the rules of English grammar. So we get 'Find it. Train it. Use it', which immediately begs the question, 'What is it?' There is no single 'it'. 'It' depends on circumstances, level of accomplishment and objective. At first all your effort, attention and training focus is on Rectification. You must find what your Rectified body feels like. With this as your guide you must relentlessly *train* your body to only express this Rectified condition. Then you can *use* your Rectified body as the tool for the next level of exploration and study which is the study of Daoyin. Again you must *find* the tracks, or spoor, of Qi as revealed in the Natural, spontaneous, preferred movements of the Rectified body. Once found they may be *trained* so that they are reinforced and strengthened. This *training* allows you to appreciate and perceive finer and finer details of movements and their accompanying sensations. These can be then *used* to allow you to progress to the final and open-ended study of Nei Gong, where once again the formula 'Find. Train. Use' applies.

So ultimately the role of the teacher in Taijiquan is considerably less than that of the student. The teacher is not so much there to teach you specific moves, techniques or forms. The teacher's job is to teach you methods to enable you to *find* whatever is relevant to your current level of development, be it Rectification, Daoyin or Nei Gong. Then the teacher should assist you with advice and suggestions as to how to *train* whatever has been found. The teacher should guide and assist you to help you avoid mistakes and unproductive dead ends. Finally the teacher will show you how to *use* whatever you have thus far *found* and *trained* either to advance to the next level or in direct application functionally and pragmatically. There is a very real sense in which an art such as Taijiquan cannot be 'taught' so much as 'learnt' by the student. Ultimately it is *your* body that is the yardstick. The teacher is at best your guide, assistant and inspiration.

PRACTISING TAIJIQUAN

Returning to nature, or Rectification of the body, to achieve 'No blocking, no wasting' is a general goal shared by many different groups for different reasons. Doctors will encourage their patients to aim for this condition because it protects from many dis-eases. Various Chinese religious orders, Taoist and Buddhist, regard this as a necessary precursor to spiritual development, the quest for 'immortality'. It is the first noticeable benefit for Taijiquan players.

Many people practise solely for this outcome. That is perfectly fine for those who do so, but we must never forget that this is really only the foundation of the art, the root for the development of the 'Quan' in Taijiquan. Even those whose interest is only in the benefits that flow from improving their 'plumbing' need the awareness of the Rectified, Three Circle and 'Non-blocked, non-wasted' model. Without it, how can they get the benefits they desire? The vast majority of practitioners in the world today practise only at the level of Rectification. This is the level that is most responsible for the positive health benefits that have become the justification for Tai Chi for Health.

Without either a good teacher or an awareness of the three-stage model Rectification, Daoyin and Nei Gong, Daoyin can become a tricky tool that may 'turn in your hand' and result in reinforcing bad habits. We could translate 'Song', from Rectification, as 'hang loose' and 'Daoyin' as 'go with the flow'. Neither of these would be incorrect, but, again, neither of them can be taken as justification for sloppiness or idleness.

In order to learn something useful we must be prepared to use our minds a little, to be thoughtful in our studies and practice. We must use our understanding, sensitivity and will to progress and we must use them in that order. We need to know what we are doing and why. Our sensitivity is used to discover the match or mis-match between our present condition and our goal. Information acquired through sensitivity plus understanding enables us to find the route from our current position to the goal. Finally, we use our will to follow that route, using sensitivity all the time so that the will is disciplined to the route, not the goal.

Chen Kung, in his discussion of the intrinsic energies of Taijiquan within his book *Taijiquan Dao Jian Kan San-Shou Ho Lun*, comments on the line in the *Taijiquan Treatise* (*Taijiquan Lun*) which says, 'After you acquire interpreting energy (Tung Jin) the more you practise the more skill you will obtain' (Olsen 1995). His comment is that 'previous to interpreting energy you must be able to perceive the one foot, then the one inch, the one tenth of an inch and finally even the one ten thousandths of an inch'. This I take to mean that we must progressively develop our awareness and sensitivity from a gross appreciation of movement, 'the one foot', to an increasingly refined perception of the finest subtleties of movement, 'the ten thousandths of an inch'. In so doing we will acquire the necessary sensitivity to finally be able to study Nei Gong. The ladder of the Six Secrets I have outlined above is a method of refining our perceptions from the gross to the fine. Somewhere along this path practitioners will find that it becomes increasingly necessary to abandon mechanical and physical descriptions and move to talk about the experience of Qi and its manipulations through 'directions of intent', the activity of the Yi. Only then can we truly talk of Nei Gong – internal or inner work.

SYLLABUS, TECHNIQUE AND METHOD

The techniques we use, the particular movements, are what makes our practice Taijiquan, rather than another form of Qi Gong, or self cultivation. A book is not a very good place to talk too much about movements and the details of movement, but that half of the door is fairly open through teachers, classes, videos and even photo books. In this book I have tried to give the other half, the not so open, to answer questions about method or stages, i.e. what is appropriate and when. To me, this means a syllabus, or description of a process of development.

Simply listing all the different forms, two person exercises, weapons and applications will not give you a syllabus for Taijiquan. The art is too holistic, self referential and embedded for such a linear list to be useful; waving your arms and legs about, with or without weapons, with or without partners, will not necessarily lead to development. Our practice must be disciplined and principled. The method I offer to remember principles is to think in terms of the stages:

• Rectification – preparing the ground

• Daoyin – learning the method

• Nei Gong – employing the method to the ground in specific order and fashion.

The relationship between these three stages and specific techniques of Taijiquan is not necessarily direct. For some students, certain practices might be more helpful at a given time, while their colleagues might need something a little different. The following table shows a more or less general programme to illustrate the relationship between the syllabus, in terms of developmental stages, and the techniques most likely to be useful.

Syllabus

Stage	Initial technique	Advanced technique
Rectification	Standing Practice, Three Circle Form	Weapons Forms, Push Hands
Daoyin	Three Circle Form, Breathing Exercises, Push Hands	Yin–Yang Form, Spiral Form, Push Weapons
Nei Gong	Yin–Yang Form, Spiral Form, Centre-Turn Form, Spiral in the Legs, Yin–Yang: Head–Hands	Da Lu, Push Hands, Two Person Form, Applications Weapons – all useful

Read down the first pair of columns to see the learning sequence for beginners. The second and third technique columns show how later techniques can feed back to further develop earlier stages and so improve accomplishment. In fact, the page is not wide enough to show the endless looping round and round that represents a life-long study and practice. Eventually 'everything' becomes 'everything else' and a point is reached where advanced practitioners really can find no other way to describe what they are doing than 'energy mechanics' – 'Qi Gong'.

INTERNAL BREATHING: NEI GONG

The 'breathing' in Taijiquan exercises a continual fascination. Whenever I visit other teachers and their students, this is the topic that raises the most questions. Everyone knows that the 'secret' of Taijiquan is in the breathing. Perhaps because breathing is something we all do continuously, people feel that they can hasten their progress by going straight to the breath. After all, it must be easier to just control my breathing than to learn all those funny moves. I'm afraid that it just does not work that way.

The last and most important 'secret' is a particular Taijiquan trick of breathing, a very simple little thing really, that is usually taught about the time of Yin–Yang: Head–Hands. It is a secret because it is such a little thing, a fine-tuning of your perception of your breathing, leading to an adjustment in your abdominal flow and pressure of breathing. It sounds clumsy in words because it is primarily motor sensations that we are talking about. It is 'reverse' breathing and the application of very developed Daoyin. The 'arm flapping' exercise in Chapter 6 (p.140), and later on used to learn 'Spiral', can also be used to learn and study the trick.

NEI GONG DAOYIN EXERCISE

Never force your breathing. I am only including this breathing trick for completeness. I do not really recommend that you try to learn this from my description. Some of you who try it may not even be able to sense the movements that I describe. In a sense you are the luckiest. You can just forget about breathing details and get on with your practice, through which it will come.

Others may feel the moves accurately and they can use the exercise, or not, as they choose. I am more concerned with people who are in between and might force their perceptions and practice, leading to damage. All I can really say is, if the exercise is not *immediately* easy to feel, grasp and practise, then *don't try* until you can learn it from a teacher.

Stand with your feet a shoulder width apart. Feet parallel, pointing straight ahead. Hang from your head, Ni Wan, and 'Song' your neck and spine to open Ming Men. Let your pelvis swing under so that Wei Lu is vertical. Sink your breathing and Qi to your lower Dantien – between Qi Hai and Ming Men. Let your knees relax 'open' and your legs become 'round', knees over toes. Raise your 'Shen' – an uncatchable spirit on the head top – and 'Song' your shoulders and the length of your arms to your fingertips. Let your elbows gently 'Song' forwards to curve your arms into a circle, fingertips touching, hands at Qi Hai.

Relax. Sink. Float. Centre your breathing and Qi in your lower Dantien. Your abdomen fills as you breathe in, empties as you breathe out. Start your arms flapping. This time direct your attention to the muscles in between the ribs. See if you can feel your diaphragm – the big sheet of muscle that separates your chest from your abdomen. Keep your breath and Qi sunk. Can you feel the lift of your ribs as the arms flap up? Can you feel your diaphragm moving with them? It can feel a bit like a piston moving up and down.

Elbows up – breathe in. Feel the ribs rising and the diaphragm sinking. Feel the breath and Qi filling your abdomen. Elbows down – breathe out. Feel the ribs and diaphragm dropping and pushing down. Feel the breath emptying the abdomen as the piston pushes, or compacts, the Qi into the lower Dantien. Feel it until you can feel all the elements simultaneously. There is no beginning and no end. Breath moves the body. The moving body is the breath. Focus on the piston. Learn the Dao of the piston so that you can use your Yi to induce that Dao when you want it.

Reduce your arm flapping but keep the piston going. Eventually the only thing you are doing is willing the piston breathing. This is then gently moving the relaxed, 'Song', round body. Breathing in 'closes' your Qi and 'inflates' your body with Qi. Breathing out 'opens' your Qi to mix with the universal Qi and packs or stores the Qi in your lower Dantien.

TESTING AND WARNINGS

The testing of this breathing is potentially rather dangerous. This is another reason why it is a late technique, rather than an early one. Both tester and testee need to have quite high levels of sensitivity and control, so as not to hurt each other. Testing involves being pushed or struck in the guts.

At the instant of contact, the testee breathes in, 'closing' the body's Qi, and 'inflating' – becoming 'round' and Yin. This will stop, and possibly reverse, the incoming Qi; when the direction of the incoming Qi stops, or reverses, breathe out. Become Yang, 'open' your Qi and focus it out at the point of contact. I do not advise this practice without a live teacher to guide and supervise safety.

Be aware that there are certain exceptions to this practice. Do not practise if you have an active abdominal disorder, the sole exception being that it can benefit certain types of constipation. Women who are actively menstruating may find this practice unpleasant or uncomfortable and it can increase blood flow in a minority of women. Should this apply to any reader, she should avoid this during her period. This practice should be completely avoided in the second trimester of pregnancy; in fact it is probably advisable to avoid it altogether if you are pregnant. Knowing the technique can apparently be very useful during birth. But if you do not know it already, it is not a very good idea to try and learn it while you actually are pregnant.

TRADITIONAL NEI GONG

Although this comes after the last of the Six Secrets, it hardly represents a completion of the development. All the previous levels are ultimately open ended in themselves and this, the entry to traditional Nei Gong, is no exception.

Very simply put, this level concerns the development of spontaneous breathing as a result of moving. You do not breathe the forms; indeed, the forms, when correctly executed, breathe you. This study is virtually impossible to present in pictures, since it is not the movements that are important now, but their effect on the breathing. The movements of the Yin phase produce inhalation; those of the Yang phase produce exhalation.

The fine-tuning of the previous levels is necessary to achieve this effect, plus the knowledge of the 'piston' of the diaphragm. I know that, anatomically, the diaphragm may not actually move that way but the idea of the 'piston' is a traditional image that I find is a useful label for my sensations.

There is a sense in which all this can be regarded as the culmination of Rectification, as well as the beginning of inner work. If the body is totally clear of blockages and wastage of Qi, then two complementary phenomena occur.

First, in static posture the natural rhythm of breathing spreads unobstructed from the centre to the four limbs. This is 'movement in stillness' and the Gong, or work, of Jing Gong or quiescent work (see p.53). It is not a deliberate work of doing but the consequence of not doing and relaxing. This is more specifically 'Song-ing', which is loosening or unbinding. It is the result of no blocking or wasting. It is the achievement also called the macrocosmic circulation of the Qi, a classically Taoist achievement, the result of not doing. By pursuing stillness, movement emerges in a classical Yin–Yang reversal.

Second, when performing forms and rounds of forms, provided the body is not blocked or wasted anywhere so that Rectification is at least minimally achieved, each move evokes breath. The source of each movement is the breath – the 'piston'. The stillness within the movements is the stillness of the Rectified, un-blocked/un-wasted, body, hence this is called Jing-Dong Gong – quiescent dynamic work (see p.55). It is the continuously emerging and developing result of the practice of Daoyin as a method.

CONCLUSION

At first, the experience and the achievement of movement in stillness will be fleeting and transitory. This feeling of the breathing moving the relaxed, stationary body, and being breathed by the movements, that is, being 'still' in the midst of movement, is difficult to achieve and maintain.

With further practice and dedicated self-study, breathing and doing forms become indistinguishable. In every move, whether during a formal practice or study session, or just the everyday movements of daily life, movement and breath are one. At least that is the goal. Few people have the persistence, opportunity or potential to progress this far. Fewer still will be able to permanently and consistently express their Qi through an unvarying link between breath and movement, regardless of being stationary or moving. Half the fun is in the permanent challenge of preserving this poised and dynamic state. The continuous expression of spirit, this continual expression of Taiji in your body, is the door to true Nei Gong and the acquisition of the marvellous advanced skills, or energies, or trained abilities, called 'Jin' in the Taijiquan literature. This entire book is only the preface to such advanced practice and development.

Appendix

Forms, Techniques and Practices

I actively teach three solo Taijiquan forms. I have studied more and will coach people who know other forms, particularly the Chen Man Ch'ing shortened, and the Big Circle Long Yang form, as introduced to the UK by Gerda Geddes in 1952.

1. The 'First Set' of Tai Chi. Very short, very gentle, suitable as an introduction and for chronic or recuperating patients.

2. Simplified (Beijing or 24-step) Tai Chi. Developed by the Sports Council of the People's Republic. Easy to learn. Most common form in the world due to its popularity in China. A 'rational' form going from simple to complex, less physically demanding to more physically demanding moves.

3. Small Circle Yang Family long form. The most demanding Yang form, with six 'secrets' or levels of development of practice. This is the basis of martial practice.

SUPPLEMENTARY FORMS AND PRACTICES

Pushing Hands

Single hand

1. fixed step

2. moving step

3. pushing leg.

Double hands

1. large circle

   a) fixed step

   b) moving step

2. small circle

   a) fixed step

   b) moving step.

Da Lu – The great pulling

1. simple form, no changes

2. four corners with changes.

Two Person Taijiquan

Essential for martial development and also very useful to refine appreciation of Yin–Yang exchanges.

Weapons Forms

These are supplementary and optional. For a person with an interest in martial art/self-defence, much of the footwork of the Yang style is developed through weapons forms. The bare hand forms generally cultivate rooting and may result in 'heavy' feet.

Sabre solo form (Taijidao).

Sword solo form, pushing swords, two person sword form (Taijijian).

Staff (Taijigun)/Spear (Taijijiang), no solo form in Yang style. Various drills and pushing spear techniques.

References

Baynes, Cary F. (trans.) (1977) *I Ching or Book of Changes: The Richard Wilhelm Translation*. London: Routledge and Kegan Paul.

Olsen, Stuart Alve (trans.) (1995) *The Intrinsic Energies of Taijiquan*. Chen kung series, vol. 2. St Paul: Dragon Door Publications.

Liang, T.T. (1977) *T'ai Chi Ch'uan for Health and Self-Defense: Philosophy and Practice*. New York: Random House.

Swain, Louis (trans.) (1999) *Fu Zhongwen: Mastering Yang Style Taijiquan*. Berkeley, CA: North Atlantic Books.

Wile, Douglas (trans.) (1983) *T'ai-chi Touchstones: Yang Family Secret Transmissions*. New York: Sweet Ch'i Press.

Bibliography

Cartmell, Tim (trans.) (2003) *A Study of Taijiquan by Sun Lutang*. Berkeley, CA: North Atlantic Books.

Chu, Wen Kuan (trans.) (1984) *Tao and Longevity: Mind–Body Transformation by Nan Huai-Chin*. Shaftesbury: Element Books.

Davis, Barbara (trans.) (2004) *The Taijiquan Classics: An Annotated Translation Including a Commentary by Chen Weiming*. Berkeley, CA: North Atlantic Books.

Feng, Gia Fu (1974) *Tai Chi, a Way of Centring and I Ching*. London: Collier Macmillan.

Frantzis, Bruce (1998) *The Power of Internal Martial Arts: Combat Secrets of Ba Gua, Tai Chi and Hsing-I*. Berkeley, CA: North Atlantic Books.

Frantzis, Bruce (2003) *The Big Book of Tai Chi: Build Health Fast in Slow Motion*. London: Thorsons.

Holbrook, Bruce (1981) *The Stone Monkey: An Alternative, Chinese-Scientific, Reality*. New York: William Morrow.

Hong, Yunxi (trans.) (1988) *14-Series Sinew-Transforming Exercises Compiled by Chang Weizhen*. Beijing: Foreign Languages Press.

Horwitz, Tem, Kimmelman, Susan and Lui, H.H. (1979) *Tai Chi Ch'uan: The Technique of Power*. London: Rider.

Huang, Wen-Shan (1979) *Fundamentals of Taijiquan*, 3rd rev. edn. Hong Kong: South Sky Books.

Jiao, Tielan (trans.) (1986) *Qigong Essentials for Health Promotion by Jiao Guorui*. Beijing: China Reconstructs Press.

Johnson, Robin (2005) *Stalking Yang Lu-Chan: Finding Your Tai Chi Body*. Santa Fe, NM: Sunstone Press.

Jou, Tsung Hwa (1982) *The Dao of Taijiquan: Way to Rejuvenation*, 3rd rev. edn. Tokyo: Tuttle Publishing.

Karcher, Stephen (2000) *Ta Chuan: The Great Treatise. The Key to Understanding the I Ching and Its Place in Your Life*. London: Carroll & Brown.

Lash, John (1989) *The Tai Chi Journey*. Shaftesbury: Element Books.

Li, Dong and Hou, Min (trans.) (1988) *Meridian Qigong Compiled and Presented by Prof Li Ding*. Beijing: Foreign Languages Press.

Liu, Zhongre (trans.) (1987) *Daoist Health Preservation Exercises*. Beijing: China Reconstructs Press.

Loupos, John (2002) *Inside Tai Chi: Hints, Tips, Training and Process for Students and Teachers*. Boston: YMMA Publication Center.

Loupos, John (2003) *Exploring Tai Chi: Contemporary Views on an Ancient Art*. Boston: YMMA Publication Center.

Lu, Shengli (2006) *Combat Techniques of Taiji, Xingyi and Bagua: Principles and Practices of Internal Martial Arts*. Berkeley, CA: Blue Snake Books.

O'Brien, Jess (ed.) (2004) *Nei Jia Quan Internal Martial Arts*. Berkeley, CA: North Atlantic Books.

Page, Michael (1988) *The Power of Ch'i: An Introduction to Chinese Mysticism and Philosophy*. Wellingborough: Aquarian Press.

Palmer, Martin (1991) *The Elements of Taoism*. Shaftesbury: Element Books.

Palmer, Martin (1997) *Yin & Yang: Understanding the Chinese Philosophy of Opposites and How to Apply It to Your Everyday Life*. London: Piatkus.

Porkert, Manfred (1985) *The Theoretical Foundations of Chinese Medicine: Systems of Correspondence*. London: MIT Press.

Wells, Marnix (2005) *Scholar Boxer: Chang Naizhou's Theory of Internal Martial Arts and the Evolution of Taijiquan*. Berkeley, CA: North Atlantic Books.

Wilder, G.D. and Ingram, J.H. (1974) *Analysis of Chinese Characters*. New York: Dover.

Wile, Douglas (1996) *Lost T'ai-chi Classics from the Late Ching Dynasty*. Albany: State University of New York Press.

Wile, Douglas (1999) *T'ai Chi's Ancestors: The Making of an Internal Art*. New York: Sweet Ch'i Press.

Wong, Kiew Kit (2001) *The Complete Book of Tai Chi Chuan: A Comprehensive Guide to the Principles and Practice*. London: Vermillion.

Wong, Kiew Kit (2002) *The Complete Book of Chinese Medicine: A Holistic Approach to Physical, Emotional and Mental Health.* Kedah: Cosmos.

Yang, Entang and Yao, Xiuqing (trans.) (1985) *Chinese Qigong Therapy Compiled by Zhang, Mingwy and Sun, Xingyuan.* Jinan: Shandong Science and Technology Press.

Zhang, Huan (2005) *Seeing beyond the Tai Chi Footprint: Sixteen Essential Principles.* Bloomington, IN: Author House.

Index